D1283539

Vestibular Function
Evaluation and Treatment

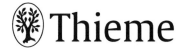 Thieme

Vestibular Function

Evaluation and Treatment

Alan Desmond, Au. D.

Blue Ridge Hearing and Balance Clinic
Bluefield, West Virginia

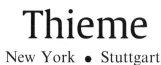

New York • Stuttgart

Thieme Medical Publishers, Inc.
333 Seventh Ave.
New York, NY 10001

Assistant Editor: Jennifer Berger
Editor: Sharon Liu
Director, Production and Manufacturing: Anne Vinnicombe
Production Editor: Becky Dille
Marketing Director: Phyllis Gold
Sales Manager: Ross Lumpkin
Chief Financial Officer: Peter van Woerden
President: Brian D. Scanlan
Compositor: Datapage International, Inc.
Printer: The Maple–Vail Book Manufacturing Group

Library of Congress Cataloging-in-Publication Data

Desmond, Alan.
Vestibular function : evaluation and treatment / Alan Desmond.
      p. ; cm.
   Includes bibliographical references and index.
   ISBN 1-58890-166-1 (TMP :alk. paper) – ISBN 3-13-136011-9 (GTV :alk. paper)
     1. Vestibluar apparatus - - Diseases - - Diagnosis. 2. Vestibular
   apparatus— Diseases— treatment. 3. Otology— Practice..
     [DNLM: 1. Vestibular Diseases— diagnosis. 2. Practice Management,
   Medical. 3. Vestibular Diseases— therapy. 4. Vestibular Function
   Tests. WV 255 D464v 2004] I. Title.
   RF260.D476 2004
   617.8'82— dc22   2003022585

Copyright © 2004 by Thieme Medical Publishers, Inc. This book, including all parts thereof, is legally protected by copyright. Any use, exploitation or commercialization outside the narrow limits set by copyright legislation, without the publisher's consent, is illegal and liable to prosecution. This applies in particular to Photostat reproduction, copying, mimeographing or duplication of any kind, translating, preparation of microfilms, and electronic data processing and storage.

Important note: Medical knowledge is ever-changing. As new research and clinical experience broaden our knowledge, changes in treatment and drug therapy may be required. The authors and editors of the material herein have consulted sources believed to be reliable in their efforts to provide information that is complete and in accord with the standards accepted at the time of publication. However, in the view of the possibility of human error by the authors, editors, or publisher, of the work herein, or changes in medical knowledge, neither the authors, editors, or publisher, nor any other party who has been involved in the preparation of this work, warrants that the information contained herein is in every respect accurate or complete, and they are not responsible for any errors or omissions or for the results obtained from·use of such information. Readers are encouraged to confirm the information contained herein with other sources. For example, readers are advised to check the product information sheet included in the package of each drug they plan to administer to be certain that the information contained in this publication is accurate and that changes have not been made in the recommended dose or in the contraindications for administration. This recommendation is of particular importance in connection with new or infrequently used drugs.

Some of the product names, patents, and registered designs referred to in this book are in fact registered trademarks or proprietary names even though specific reference to this fact is not always made in the text. Therefore, the appearance of a name without designation as proprietary is not to be construed as a representation by the publisher that it is in the public domain.

Printed in the United States of America

5 4 3 2

TMP ISBN 1-58890-166-1
GTV ISBN 3 13 136011 9

Contents

Foreword

The dizzy patient presents a unique diagnostic dilemma. With so many etiologies to consider, the patient is best served by a team of health care practitioners working together rather than by individual specialists, each with their own particular strengths and inherent limitations. This "balance center" concept is the basis for Alan Desmond's book, *Vestibular Function: Evaluation and Treatment*.

Written as an introductory text, the author takes the reader through a thoughtful explanation of the nature and variety of balance disorders and the treatment options for each, combined with some excellent practical advice regarding the establishment of a multidisciplinary balance team. Most important, emphasis is on the appropriate role for each member of the team—physician, audiologist, therapist, technician—to achieve the optimal outcome for the patient.

I have followed Dr. Desmond's work throughout its entire course, from conception to publication, when it began as a dissertation for his doctoral degree. Throughout its development, he has been open to suggestion and even criticism for the sake of a more precise and readable work. I am honored to write this foreword and to praise the finished product, which can serve as a valuable springboard for those interested in embarking along this lifelong path of learning and discovery that is necessary to caring for these challenging patients. It is hoped that we will all learn to work together within the scope of our own training for the common good of the dizzy patient.

I wish the best to those who read this work and hope you all will gain the same satisfaction in this field of medicine that I have enjoyed over the last 18 years!

Joel A. Goebel, M.D., F.A.C.S.
Professor and Vice Chairman
Director, Hearing and Balance Center
Department of Otolaryngology–Head and Neck Surgery
Washington University School of Medicine
Saint Louis, Missouri

Preface

An Introduction to the Evaluation and Treatment of Vestibular Dysfunction

The process of developing scientific truths is often the combination of meticulous research and serendipitous observation. The acceptance of those truths into standard practice typically requires replicable evidence; a need for a "better way"; and advocates for change who are persistent, committed, and stubborn enough to differ publicly from the established norm. A quote by Max Planck (mined from Dr. Alec Salt's Cochlear Fluids Lab Web page www.oto.wustl.edu/cochlea/) highlights the struggle of proposing an alternative to conventional thinking: "A new scientific truth does not triumph by convincing its opponents and making them see the light, but rather because its opponents eventually die and a new generation grows up that are familiar with it."

The development of current techniques used in the evaluation and treatment of vestibular dysfunction has a rich heritage of accidental discovery. One of the first published reports regarding nystagmus was the observation of Purkinje who, in the early 1800s, noticed postrotary nystagmus in mental patients. The rotary apparatus at the time was a large cage suspended from a rope. The cage was manually rotated to induce nausea (and a more passive nature, it was hoped) in violent patients (Barany, 1916). Postrotary nystagmus is still used as a measure of sensitivity in contemporary vestibular testing (Furman & Cass, 1996).

Robert Barany, who won the Nobel Prize for his vestibular research in 1916, first began to examine the effects of caloric stimulation of the ear canal after several of his patients complained of dizziness following irrigation intended to remove cerumen from the ear canal (Barany, 1916). Currently, caloric irrigation is the mainstay of vestibular evaluation.

One of the most dramatic recent developments in the treatment of vestibular dysfunction, "Canalith Repositioning Maneuvers for Benign Positional Vertigo," began when Brandt and Daroff (1980) designed exercises they thought promoted central compensation by repeated exposure to the offending position. They soon realized that the rapid rate of recovery could not be explained by central nervous system habituation and suspected "dispersion of otolithic debris from the cupula."

Not all early observations have withstood the test of time. Bach (not the composer) in the late 1800s noted that nystagmus patterns differed among individuals following similar rotational stimulus. He observed that "one almost invariably finds pronounced nystagmus in normal persons of cultured status, and in sensitive easily excited and nervous persons, while on the contrary (one finds) often no nystagmus at all or only slight nystagmus in stupid, indifferent and phlegmatic personalities" (Bach, 1894).

With the advent of computer-based diagnostic capabilities and nearly instant Internet access to current research, continued use of "conventional wisdom" in the evaluation and treatment of vestibular patients must be superseded by an evidence-based approach. The most critical aspect of improving the likelihood of successful treatment for vestibular disorders lies in the acceptance of evidence-based approaches to treatment and access to properly trained practitioners. This book hopes to provide assistance toward both these goals.

References

Bach, L. (1894). Ueber Kunstlich erzeugeten nystagmus bei normalen individen und bei taubstummen, Beitrag zur physiologie des ohrlabyrinthes. *Arch F Augenh 30,* 10.

Barany, R. (1916). Some new methods for functional testing of the vestibular *apparatus and the cerebellum.* Nobel lectures 1901–1921. Amsterdam-London-New York: Elsevier.

Brandt, T., & Daroff, R. (1980). Physical therapy for benign paroxysmal positional vertigo. Arch Otolaryyngol, 106, 484-485.

Furman, J. M., & Cass, S. P. (1996). Laboratory evaluation: Electronystagmography and rotational testing. In Baloh, R.W., & Halmagyi, G. M. (Eds.), *Disorders of the vestibular system*. New York: Oxford University Press.

Acknowledgements

Many people have contributed to this project, both directly and indirectly. Professionally, Dr. Michael Valente provided invaluable editing, advice, and encouragement, and saw this project through from conception to publication. Dr. Joel Goebel and Dr. Ted Glattke contributed many hours and, more importantly, many great ideas as the project developed. Dr. Holly Hosford-Dunn has been a long time friend and mentor, and is largely responsible for my growth as an audiologist.

I want to thank my colleagues and staff at Blue Ridge Hearing and Balance Clinic. My partners of more than twenty years, Dr. Lee Smith and Dr. Robert Jones, and my colleague in the balance clinic, Dr. R. Brian Collie, played a large role in the development and growth of the clinic. A special thanks to my staff, particularly Donna Johnson and Tara Minnix. I am fortunate to be surrounded by a group of such smart and dedicated people.

From a personal perspective, my parents, Louis and Margaret Desmond, have been steadfast supporters even when my focus and effort level may have been less than steadfast. They taught me to work hard and "do the right thing" by example. My wife and daughters, Jaletta, Jocelyn, and Julia, provided inspiration, demonstrated patience, and gave needed mental breaks during the book writing process.

The Need for Balance Centers

Dizziness and dysequilibrium are common complaints in both the general adult and the geriatric populations. The patient who complains of dizziness often presents a diagnostic and management dilemma to the attending physician, audiologist, or physical therapist. Dizziness is a symptom that cannot be quantified, and a lengthy case history is needed to understand the sensation the patient is describing.

The cause of dizziness can range from benign self-limiting conditions to potentially life-threatening conditions. Dizziness and dysequilibrium can occur from disruptions in one or more of the sensory systems responsible for balance or from inaccurate integration and central processing of information received from these sensory systems. Dizziness could be the result of an identifiable pathology or a combination of any number of subclinical pathologies. The cause may be otologic, neurologic, cardiovascular, psychiatric, orthopedic, ophthalmologic, or none of these. The *Physicians Desk Reference* lists dizziness, lightheadedness, or related complaints as side effects for nearly 1000 medications (Smith, 1990). Ironically, many medications used to treat dizziness list dizziness as a common side effect.

The attending health care provider (HCP)[1] must make management decisions based on the patient's history, physical examination, and the HCP's own knowledge of the various causes of dizziness as well as the likelihood of particular pathologies based on epidemiologic information.

Epidemiology Studies

Epidemiologic data typically include reviews of the incidence of complaints of dizziness in a general medical practice or reviews of diagnostic results in a population of dizzy patients consulting a specialty clinic. Only recently has the

---

[1] The term *health care provider* (HCP) is used throughout this book. Although certain activities fall squarely and solely in the realm of one specialty, the term *HCP* has been used to avoid any inference of what specialty should (or should not) be involved in a particular activity. Scope of Practice will be discussed in Chapter 7.

issue of the prevalence of unreported bothersome dizziness in the general population been explored. The outcomes of all such studies are inevitably influenced by the experimental design of the study. Sloane and Dallara (1999) point out that most studies tend to enroll patients with an isolated primary complaint of dizziness or those with chronic or recurrent symptoms. They also note that many studies focus on establishing a final diagnosis and give little attention to outcomes, symptom resolution, or reduction in disability. Epidemiologic studies should be viewed as "part of the puzzle," but the reader is advised not to draw conclusions from any one study.

Prevalence

General Population

Various reports list dizziness as one of the most common complaints in the primary care setting. Nazareth, Yardley, Owen, and Luxon (1999) report that 4% of patients 18 to 65 years of age who consult a general practice medical office report persistent symptoms of dizziness and that 3% consider their dizziness "severely incapacitating." Yardley, Owen, Nazareth, and Luxon (1998) speculate that the incidence of bothersome dizziness might be underreported if only those patients seeking medical assistance were included. They performed a survey of a random sample of patients in general practice medical offices with no selection criteria as to why they had visited the medical office. They found that more than 20% of the general population aged 18 to 65 reported experiencing dizziness within the previous month. Half of those (or 10% of the total) reported some degree of handicap associated with dizziness.

A follow-up study of the same group 18 months later (Nazareth et al., 1999) concluded that 29% of respondents reporting dizziness were more handicapped by their symptoms 18 months later. Only 22% had consulted with their physician during the 18 months since the previous study. Their final conclusion was that dizziness is much more common, chronic, and debilitating than previous reports suggested.

Older Population

The prevalence of dizziness in the general population is high, but its reported incidence increases in the aged population. Dizziness was the third most common complaint recorded in a 3-year study of common symptoms of 1000 internal medicine outpatients with a mean age of 59.3 years. Only chest pain and fatigue were noted more frequently in this group (Kroenke & Mangelsdorff, 1989). As the mean age of the patients increases, the reported incidence of dizziness also increases. Sloane, Blazer, and George (1989) report that "18.3% of adults age 60 and older are estimated to have suffered dizziness significant enough to result in a physician visit, taking a medication, or interfering with normal activities 'a lot' during the past year." Of particular significance is the fact that in persons over the age of 75, dizziness is the most common reason for a physician visit (Koch & Smith, 1985).

Persistent Symptoms

Not only is the incidence of dizziness high in relation to many other patient complaints, but the symptoms are frequently persistent and ongoing. Kroenke et al. (1992) reported on a group of 100 patients with a mean age of 62 years whose reason for initial consultation was a complaint of dizziness. More than 70% of these patients did not have a resolution of symptoms at 2-week follow-up. In a follow-up study, Kroenke, Lucas, Rosenberg, Scherokman, and Herbers (1994) reported on the 1-year outcomes in the same group of patients. They found that "The dizziness resolved for 18 patients, whereas the status improved for 37, stayed the same for 32, and worsened for 11, with two patients lost to follow up."

Aging Population

Most HCPs are aware of the "graying of America" and its impact on the number of people requiring medical attention over the next few decades. According to the U.S. Census Bureau, the elderly population (defined as 65 years and older) will more than double in the first half of the twenty-first century (www.census.gov/socdemo). This is the fastest growing segment of society, and by 2030 may represent 20% of the total U.S. population. The "very old" group (85+) is expected to quadruple during the same period (Shapiro, 1999). These statistics are likely the result of improved nutrition and medical care. Life expectancy in 1900 was 47 years; by 1991 it had extended to 76 years (U.S. Census Bureau, 1999). The average education and income levels of the geriatric population are also rising rapidly. It may be assumed, then, that the demand for effective treatments for dizziness will increase as the current population ages.

Etiology

Several studies have been performed to determine the probable cause of dizziness in a selected group of individuals (Colledge et al., 1996; Katsarkis, 1994; Kroenke, et al., 1992; Lawson, Fitzgerald, Birchall, Aldren, & Kenny, 1999; Sloane, 1989). These studies differ both in the group studied (typically by age) and the group completing the study (primary care versus specialty dizziness clinic). It would seem that data obtained by specialty clinics would be influenced by the fact that if a patient were referred to an otology- or neurology-based clinic for evaluation, someone (either the patient or the primary care physician) has already suspected that the cause of dizziness may be otologic or neurologic in nature.

Vestibular Disorders

Seeking to determine the most common causes of dizziness, Kroenke et al. (1992) performed a detailed questionnaire, physical examination, vestibular evaluation by a neuro-ophthalmologist, laboratory tests including electrocardiograph (ECG), audiometry, and structured psychiatric interview on 100 patients presenting to four different outpatient settings (internal medicine, walk-in, emergency room, and neurology) with a chief complaint of dizziness. Only patients whose dizziness persisted at 2 weeks after the initial consultation were included in the study. They found that "Primary causes of dizziness included vestibular disorders (54 patients), psychiatric disorders (16 patients), presyncope (six patients), dysequilibrium (two patients), and hyperventilation (one patient); dizziness was multicausal in 13 patients and of unknown cause in eight patients." The mean age of these 100 patients was 61.7 years, and the group selected was fairly heterogeneous in respect to the site of presentation.

Benign Paroxysmal Positional Vertigo

When discussing the etiology of complaints of dizziness, one must consider the possibility that some patients are incorrectly categorized as a result of possible misdiagnosis. Katsarkas (1994), seeking to identify leading causes of dizziness, performed a retrospective study of 1194 patients (mean age, 75.4 years) presenting to a dizziness clinic. All patients underwent a neurologic examination; however, additional studies such as electronystagmography (ENG), audiometry, and neuroimaging were performed "depending on diagnostic requirements." He reported that more than one third of these patients were found to have "confirmed or strongly suspected" benign paroxysmal positional vertigo (BPPV) and that more than half were suspected of peripheral vestibular pathology. Twenty-two percent of this subject group showed symptoms that were "non-specific, and the diagnosis was uncertain."

Katsarkis (1994) states that the "Syndromes of vestibular dysfunction are frequently misdiagnosed or dizziness is just attributed to aging," and "it is strongly suspected that paroxysmal positional vertigo is frequently misdiagnosed as vascular disease in advanced age." Li, Li, Epley, and Weinberg (2000) also suggest that BPPV is frequently misdiagnosed in both the primary care and specialty clinic setting.

Vestibular Pathology

Colledge et al. (1996) also found a high prevalence of abnormal vestibular test results in a group of older people (mean age, 76.3 years). Their interpretation of these data, however, was that vestibular pathology was overestimated as a cause of dizziness because they found no significant difference in results of ENG between dizzy patients and their asymptomatic control group. Because they did not specify what abnormalities were noted on ENG, and the ENG protocol they describe examines both peripheral and central pathologies, it is difficult to interpret these findings. They also report no significant differences between dizzy patients and the control group in blood tests, ECG, and magnetic resonance imaging (MRI) of the head and neck.

Hypertension

Sloane (1989) reviewed the results of the national ambulatory care survey (Table 1–1), which indicates that hypertension is the most frequent diagnosis among

Table 1–1. Most Common Primary Diagnoses Associated with a Chief Complaint of Dizziness

Physician Category	Chief Complaint	Percent
Primary care		
25–54 yr (*n* = 17)	Hypertension	17.0
	Labyrinthitis	17.0
	Dizziness, unspecified	13.4
	Hypoglycemia	3.5
55–74 yr (*n* = 232)	Hypertension	27.1
	Dizziness, unspecified	14.2
	Labyrinthitis	11.2
	Diabetes mellitus	3.9
75+ yr (*n* = 128)	Hypertension	13.3
	Coronary atherosclerosis	6.4
	Dizziness, unspecified	7.8
	Labyrinthitis	7.0
Specialist practice		
25–54 yr (*n* = 124)	Dizziness, unspecified	11.3
	Meniere's disease	6.5
	Benign positional vertigo	6.5
	Hypertension	6.5
55–74 yr (*n* = 136)	Dizziness, unspecified	11.0
	Hypertension	10.3
	Labyrinthitis	8.1
	Meniere's disease	5.1
75+ yr (*n* = 59)	Dizziness, unspecified	25.4
	Labyrinthitis	6.8
	Hypertension	6.8
	Unspecified cerebrovascular disease	6.8

In adults aged 25 years and older by age category, primary care physician, and specialists. National Ambulatory Medical Care Survey (NSMCS) combined data 1981 and 1985, unweighted.

Reprinted with permission from Sloane, P. D., Dallara J., Roach, C., Bailey, K. E., Mitchell, M., & McNutt, R. (1994). Management of dizziness in primary care. *J Am Board Fam Pract, 7,* 1–8.

patients complaining of dizziness. He points out that the "prevalence of hypertension in the general population approaches that among patients with dizziness" and suggests that physicians "may be biased toward a so-called hard diagnosis such as hypertension" to explain the patient's complaint of dizziness. He suggests, therefore, that hypertension might be misdiagnosed as the cause of dizziness in some patients when the real cause is unknown.

Cardiovascular Diagnosis

Lawson et al. (1999) performed extensive evaluations on a group of older subjects (mean age, 74 years), including audiometry, ENG, and postural stability assessment as well as ECG, 24-hour cardiac monitoring, and orthostatic blood pressure measurements. Their results differed substantially from those of Kroenke et al. (1992) and Katsarkas (1994) in that "Twenty eight percent had a cardio-vascular diagnosis, 18% had a peripheral vestibular disorder, 14% had a central neurological disorder, 18% had more than one diagnosis, and 22% had no attributable cause of symptoms identified." It is clear that epidemiology studies are often affected by examiner bias, incorrect diagnosis, and choice of diagnostic tests used. As in any type of statistical analysis, a larger data pool will increase the likelihood of accurate findings.

Combined Literature Review

Kroenke, Hoffman, and Einstadter (2000) performed a literature review of 12 articles related to etiology of dizziness (some noted previously). In combining those reports, they found the following: "Dizziness was attributed to a peripheral vestibulopathy in 44% of patients, a central vestibulopathy in 11%, psychiatric causes in 16%, other conditions in 26%, and unknown cause in 13%. Certain causes were relatively uncommon, including cerebrovascular disease (6%), cardiac arrhythmia (1.5%), and brain tumor (< 1%)."

Lord, Clark, and Webster (1991) and Tinnetti, Williams, and Gill (2000) approached the subject of dizziness in the older patients from a different perspective. Lord et al. (1991), in examining a group of older persons (mean age, 82.7 years) found that decreased peripheral sensation (in the lower extremities) "is the most important sensory system in the maintenance of static postural stability." They believed this was the result of "reduced tactile sensitivity, joint position and vibration sense, and reduced quadriceps and ankle dorsiflexion strength." Tinetti et al. (2000) suggest that dizziness in older patients may be a geriatric syndrome involving multiple causative factors and did not find any single factor that could be blamed in most cases. It appears that there is great subjectivity in providing a diagnosis and that the diagnosis is clearly influenced by which tests are chosen for a particular study. A notable weakness of each of these studies is the lack of any type of rotational testing, which has been shown to identify vestibular pathology in patients with otherwise normal vestibular evaluations (Desmond & Touchette, 1998; Saddat, O'Leary, Pulec, & Kitano, 1995; Shepard, Telian, & Smith-Wheelock, 1996.)

Quality of Life

Although data published in primary care journals indicate a low incidence of mortality and institutionalization associated with complaints of dizziness (Boult, Murphy, Sloane, Mor, & Drone, 1991; Sloane, 1989), recent reports have shown a correlation between dizziness and functional decline, disability, and decreased quality of life. It has been reported that dizziness has a greater impact on quality of life and functional abilities than many other chronic conditions: Grimby and

Rosenhall (1995) report that when comparing older patients with dizziness with older patients without dizziness, the dizzy patients consistently rate their quality of life as being lower and consume significantly more medications. They also report a higher frequency of falls in patients with dizziness.

Using the Short Form Health Survey (SF-36), a generic health status assessment used in more than 40 countries (Ware, Phillips, Benson, & Adamczyk, 1996), Enloe and Shields (1997) found that patients with vestibular disorders had lower scores for health-related quality of life than does the general population. Significantly, they also found that these scores improved after 6 to 8 weeks of vestibular rehabilitation.

Behavioral Changes

Fear of becoming dizzy is a frequently noted complaint of patients with chronic or episodic dizziness, and it can frequently lead to changes in a patient's behavior. Newman and Jacobson (1993) offer the following explanation for the dramatic effect even intermittent dizziness can have on the daily life of the affected patient:

"Frank spells of vertigo in public may cause patients to change their occupation (e.g., a painter who must climb tall ladders), restrict their mobility (a person may stop driving for fear of endangering the life of another because of the unpredictability of the onset of episodes of dizziness), cease leisure activities with friends or family (e.g., for fear of ruining an otherwise pleasurable activity by becoming suddenly or violently ill), stop necessary household activities such as food shopping (e.g., due to the possibility of becoming ill and incapacitated in a public place), and become housebound in the most severe cases. It has been our observation that unlike other disorders such as hearing loss that might require numerous negative experiences to cause a change in behavior, dizziness and vertigo attacks may need to occur only a few times before a patient might change his or her normal daily routines. Unlike other disorders such as tinnitus and hearing loss that are more or less constant, vertigo is usually unpredictable and when it occurs leaves the patient with a feeling of helplessness." (Newman & Jacobson, 1993, p. 363)

Impact of Dizziness

Honrubia, Bell, Harris, Baloh, and Fisher (1996) explored self-rated quality of life for specific vestibular pathologies. They found that BPPV had the lowest impact on quality of life compared with other conditions, such as Meniere's disease or other peripheral or central vestibulopathy. Although not discussed in the article, one must wonder whether the predictable nature of BPPV reduces the fear and anxiety associated with episodic vertigo.

These authors also report that "the physicians' estimation of the impact of dizziness on the patients' quality of life was different from the patients' opinion," with patients reporting a greater impact. They also found a higher prevalence of anxiety and depression in their pool of dizzy patients than would be found in the general population, and they suggest that patients expressing fear and distress related to their dizziness may need professional counseling. Other reports also support this suggestion, showing that patients with complaints of dizziness have higher levels of anxiety, a higher incidence of panic disorder, and a greater likelihood of agoraphobia and social avoidance behaviors than do non-dizzy subjects (Alvord, 1991; Clark, Hirsch, Smith, Furman, & Jacob, 1994; Sullivan et al., 1993).

Management Trends

Even though the diagnostic capabilities and treatment options available to vestibular patients have increased dramatically in the last two decades, most patients complaining of dizziness do not have access to trained vestibular specialists. This lack of access is the result both of geographic considerations (lack of a local facility) and resistance or unfamiliarity by the medical community to accept more current treatment techniques. It has been reported that physicians in some specialties (in the case of the quoted study, cardiology) often rely exclusively on information learned in medical school (Ghali, Saits, Sargious, & Hershman, 1999) or on information from "textbooks, which have been shown to lag in their treatment recommendations by as much as fifteen years" (Antman, Lau, Kupelnick, Mosteller, & Chalmers, 1992).

Specialist and Primary Care Physician Visits

Patients are more likely to seek medical advice when they are unclear as to the cause of their symptoms (Clark, Sullivan, & Katon, 1993). Because dizziness has been notoriously difficult to diagnose, imagine the confusion of the patient in selecting which specialist to consult when experiencing these symptoms. Most patients choose to consult their primary care physician (PCP) rather than seeking the advice of a specialist directly. (It should be noted that some managed care health plans mandate this.) In fact, fewer than 10% of dizzy patients are evaluated by an otologist or neurologist (Table 1–2). More than 70% of patients complaining of dizziness are seen by either general or internal medicine

Table 1–2. Proportion of Patients Aged 25+ Seen by Various Physician Specialists Because of Dizziness, United States, 1985

Physician Specialist	Percent
General Practitioners/Family Practice	44.3
General internists	22.6
Other internal medicine subspecialists	6.2
Otorhinolaryngologists	6.2
Cardiologists	5.5
Other	4.5
General surgeons	4.3
Neurologists	3.6
Surgical subspecialists (including OB/GYN)	2.8

NAMCS, National Ambulatory Medical Care Survey; OB/GYN, obstetrics/gynecology. Reprinted with permission from Sloane, P. D., (1989). Dizziness in primary care: results from the national ambulatory medical care survey. *J Fam Pract 29*, 33–38.

practitioners (Sloane, 1989). Because these specialties represent only 42.1% of all ambulatory patient visits, a grossly disproportionate number of dizzy patients are being managed by primary care physicians (McElmore and Delozier, 1985; Sloane, 1989).

Primary Care Approach to Management

Several articles have explored the diagnostic and treatment approaches used in many primary care offices. Sloane (1989) reports that of 531 adults complaining of dizziness, 89% were prescribed medication, most frequently meclizine. Between 1 and 2% were hospitalized for nonvestibular conditions and 4.4% were referred on to specialists. Most were provided a return appointment.

A prospective 6-month study reported in 1994 (Sloane et al., 1994) revealed the management strategies used by PCPs when evaluating a patient with a complaint of dizziness. These strategies are listed in Table 1–3. Even though the most common initial impression by the physician and final diagnosis were otologic, only 3 of 140 patients were referred for otologic studies (two for audiograms and one for an ENG examination). More than 10% were referred for neuroimaging or vascular studies, and, as noted in Table 1–3, more than 61% received a prescription for medication, again most commonly meclizine.

These management trends indicate that PCPs appear to be more focused on potentially life-threatening conditions as opposed to the patient's quality of life. This is consistent with the findings of Honrubia et al. (1996) that physicians tend to underestimate the effect dizziness can have on quality of life. A quote from the study "Management of Dizziness in Primary Care" (Sloane et al., 1994) may provide some insight as to the primary care approach: "Physicians tend to treat more conservatively the more classic symptoms of vertigo, which often have self limiting causes, and to conduct more investigation when neurologic or cardiologic diagnosis was suspected."

Table 1–3. Management Strategies (*n* = 140) Used by Primary Care Providers in Evaluating a Patient with a Complaint of Dizziness

Treatment Strategy	Percent
Office laboratory testing	33.6
Advanced testing	11.4
Referral to a specialist	9.3
Medication	61.3
Observation	71.8
Reassurance	41.6
Behavioral recommendations	15.0

Reprinted with permission from Sloane, P. D., Dallara J., Roach, C., Bailey, K. E., Mitchell, M., & McNutt, R. (1994). Management of dizziness in primary care. *J Am Board Fam Pract, 7,* 1–8.

Review of Management Decisions in Primary Care

A point-by-point examination of the management decisions listed in Table 1–3 indicates that available data do not support these decisions as being effective approaches to the dizzy patient.

Office Laboratory Testing

One third of the patients in the aforementioned study by Sloane et al. (1994) underwent office laboratory tests. Kroenke et al. (1992) performed comprehensive medical and neuro-otological evaluations as well as structured psychiatric interviews on 100 patients consulting primary care settings with complaints of persistent dizziness. Laboratory tests consisted of "complete blood count (CBC), a 20-item screening chemistry panel, thyroid function tests, and EKG evaluation." Their conclusion was that these laboratory tests "were not useful in establishing a cause" for the patients' complaints.

Stewart et al. (1999) performed a retrospective review of 192 patients seen at a specialty clinic for the specific complaint of vertigo (as opposed to the more vague complaint of dizziness). Physicians at the clinic performed a battery of tests that included audiometry, ENG, posturography, MRI of the head, and laboratory tests, including urinalysis, erythrocyte sedimentation rate, antinuclear antibody test, fluorescent treponemal antibody test, and thyroid function test. In establishing a diagnosis they found that "blood tests may have a significant diagnostic efficiency in certain patients, although as a routine diagnostic test in patients with vertigo, we found that blood tests were not cost effective." Colledge et al. (1996) report that "no differences were found between the two groups (older dizzy versus older non-dizzy control) in the results of blood tests," which included "blood count, erythrocyte sedimentation rate, urea and electrolyte concentrations, random glucose concentration, triglyceride concentration, and cholesterol concentration and for performance of liver and thyroid function tests."

Advanced Testing

IMAGING

"Balance disorders are common, while brain tumors are rare. An isolated balance disorder is thus rarely the presenting symptom of a brain tumor, and some physicians, particularly in countries infested with lawyers, worry about missing a brain tumor." (Hirose & Halmagyi, 1996). This quote by Hirose and Halmagyi (1996), both practicing neurologists outside the United States (Japan and Australia, respectively), eloquently sums up the trend of ordering cranial MRI scans for patients presenting with dizziness, despite data indicating this to be an extremely ineffective use of health care dollars. Sloane et al. (1994) report that 11.4% of patients complaining of dizziness at the primary care level were scheduled for "advanced testing." One third of those patients were referred for CT scan or MRI studies of the head.

Colledge et al. (1996) performed cranial MRI scans on 125 older dizzy patients and 86 control subjects. They report "abnormalities were widespread and present in most subjects regardless of group. Eighty-seven (70%) dizzy subjects and 57 (66%) control subjects had facet joint degeneration, 105 (84%) dizzy subjects and 70 (81%) controls had cerebellar atrophy, and 85 (68%) and 64 (74%), respectively, had white matter lesions in the cerebral hemisphere." These findings would suggest that MRI alone does not provide useful information about the diagnosis of dizziness.

Day et al. (1990) report that MRI scanning is the test of choice when neuroimaging of the older dizzy patient is indicated. They state, "Vascular insufficiency of the brainstem (often loosely referred to as vertebro-basilar insufficiency) is widely considered to be one of the more common factors in the elderly" and that "MRI carries substantial advantages in imaging the posterior fossa and brain stem areas that are often poorly demonstrated on conventional CT transmission." They reviewed cranial MRI scans of 20 older patients (mean age, 82 years) complaining of dizziness and nine similarly aged control patients. Consistent with the previously mentioned study by Colledge et al. (1996), Day et al. (1990) found abnormalities in nearly all subjects from both groups but found no significant differences. They conclude that cranial MRI scanning is not helpful in the diagnosis of dizziness for most older patients.

Richard Prass, MD, a practicing neuro-otologist at Atlantic Coast Ear Specialists *(www.earaces.com)*, reports that 43% of 369 consecutive patients referred for dizziness had previously been referred for MRI scanning. He performed a review of all MRI films and found that "four percent of these studies were read as abnormal, and one (less than 1%) was considered to be helpful in diagnosing the patient's complaints."

IMAGING COSTS

Gizzi, Riley, & Molinari (1996), make the point that conditions such as cerebrovascular disease, demyelinating disease, and intracranial masses typically present with central nervous system (CNS) findings in addition to the complaint of dizziness. Diagnosis of otologic causes of dizziness, such as Meniere's disease, labyrinthitis, or BPPV, is typically not helped by imaging studies. They postulate that MRI scanning for patients with no CNS signs is only helpful in the evaluation for acoustic neuroma and that this diagnosis in the presence of symmetrical hearing is rare. Based on their statistical analysis regarding epidemiology of acoustic neuroma, they report the probability of a positive finding in a dizzy patient with no CNS signs and symmetrical hearing to be one in 9307. Based on the average cost of a MRI scan with contrast, which is estimated at $1200 (Bauch, 1992), the cost of finding one acoustic neuroma in this population would be $11,168,400. When the criteria for scanning is simply changed to include only patients with asymmetrical hearing loss, the probability of a positive finding increases to one in 638, representing a projected cost of $765,600.

LOW-COST ALTERNATIVE IMAGING TECHNIQUES

It is acknowledged that there are reasons other than searching for an acoustic neuroma to perform MRI scanning on dizzy patients. MRI scanning can provide evidence of multiple sclerosis, mass lesion, and cerebral atrophy or ischemia, although less costly screening MRI examinations such as fast-spin echo are not sensitive to these conditions. Most CNS lesions related to dizziness are located in the cerebellum or brainstem (Ojala, Ketonen, & Palo, 1988), which are not examined with fast-spin echo technique.

The yield of MRI scanning for dizziness increases dramatically when patients are selected based on the results of preliminary examinations or clinical suspicion of CNS involvement. As mentioned earlier, asymmetrical sensorineural hearing loss and persistent unilateral tinnitus are clinical indicators for performing imaging studies to rule out auditory nerve pathology. Ojala et al. (1988) used history, ENG, auditory-evoked potentials, electroencephalography (EEG), and cerebrospinal fluid studies to screen patients before ordering MRI scanning. They found that 40% of scanned patients had findings relevant to their complaints of dizziness. Ojala et al. (1988) also suggest that the areas of the brain most likely to demonstrate lesions causing dizziness are better viewed through MRI than CT scanning.

Referral to a Specialist

Bird, Beynon, Prevost, and Bagulry (1998) reviewed the referral patterns of PCPs in England. In their retrospective review of the management of 503 patients presenting with dizziness, they found that, according to published best practice patterns, 17% of management decisions were inappropriate and the "major failing was not referring appropriate patients." Their conclusion is as follows: "Patients with chronic symptoms of dizziness, particularly the elderly, are under referred for specialist consultation and, therefore, do not have access to appropriate treatment regimes. This suggests a need for further training of GPs and evaluation of therapeutic needs of elderly dizzy patients."

Medication

The previously mentioned study by Sloane et al. (1994) states that 61.3% of patients complaining of dizziness are given medication by the attending primary care doctor. The medication most often used was meclizine, a vestibular suppressant. Ideally, medication used to suppress symptoms would be used only during the acute stage following vestibular insult. During the acute phase of vestibular dysfunction (typically lasting 3 to 5 days) vestibular suppressants are helpful in reducing the activity in the vestibular nuclei and cerebellum (Shepard et al., 1996). It is the tonic asymmetry in activity in these areas that creates the acute symptoms of vestibular-induced vertigo. For natural or therapeutically enhanced compensation to take place, the brain eventually must be made aware that an asymmetry exists (Desmond, 2000).

USE OF VESTIBULAR SUPPRESSANT MEDICATION

Although specialists in the area of vestibular rehabilitation generally agree that vestibular compensation is inhibited by the use of vestibular or CNS sedative medications (Brandt, 1991; Shepard, Telian, & Smith-Wheelock, 1990; Zee, 1985), the literature suggests that these types of medications are usually used when a patient arrives in the primary care setting with the complaint of dizziness, vertigo, or imbalance. Of these patients, 61 to 89% receive some type of medication following their initial visit. The most commonly used medication is meclizine (Antivert) (Burke, 1995; Sloane, 1989; Sloane, et al., 1994). Li et al. (2000) report that 90% of patients subsequently diagnosed with BPPV were given meclizine before receiving a correct diagnosis.

Appropriate treatment following the acute phase would encourage activity to promote central compensation (Desmond, 2000). Additionally, some patients describing imbalance have normal vestibular function and may be experiencing imbalance or dysequilibrium from another cause. *Dizziness* is a vague term that can mean different things to different people. A recent study (Tinnetti et al., 2000) reports that of older patients complaining of dizziness, only 25% were describing rotary vertigo. On further questioning, about 75% described their dizziness as unsteadiness, dysequilibrium, loss of balance, or presyncopal lightheadedness. Although the etiology of these complaints was not obtained, we know that BPPV is the most common cause of vertigo, and dysequilibrium and unsteadiness can be the result of vestibular or nonvestibular pathology. Patients with dysequilibrium or unsteadiness may actually experience greater symptoms because suppressant medications may hinder the function of the vestibular apparatus at a time when the patient may be most dependent on it.

STUDIES USING MECLIZINE

Kroenke, Arrington, and Mangelsdorff (1990) report that only 31% of patients receiving medication for dizziness found it helpful. In addition, considering the frequency that meclizine (Antivert) is prescribed for dizziness, it has been the subject of remarkably few studies to evaluate its effectiveness and side effects. In 1972 a randomized, double-blind crossover study indicated that meclizine had a greater effect than a placebo on diminishing symptoms and signs of vertigo of vestibular origin (Cohen & deJong, 1972). Scopolamine has been more effective than meclizine in treating the symptoms of motion sickness (Dahl, Offer-Ohlson, Lillevoid, & Sandvik, 1984). No known studies have indicated that meclizine provides any benefit for complaints of dysequilibrium, imbalance, or lightheadedness. The *Physicians Desk Reference (www.PDR.net)* (2001) reports that indications for the use of meclizine are "effective: management of nausea and vomiting, and dizziness associated with motion sickness," and "possibly effective: management of vertigo associated with diseases affecting the vestibular system." Adverse reactions are listed as: "Drowsiness, dry mouth and, on rare occasions, blurred vision have been reported" (Fig. 1–1).

In the 1960s and mid-1980s, two contradictory anecdotal case reports were published. Kutscher, Zegarelli, Hyman, and Tovell (1966) described a case of a woman taking meclizine for several years with no reported or measurable side

ANTIVERT® TABLETS   ℞
[ăn 'ti-vert ˘]
(12.5 mg meclizine HCl)
ANTIVERT®/25 TABLETS   ℞
(25 mg meclizine HCl)
ANTIVERT®/50 TABLETS   ℞
(50 mg meclizine HCl)

DESCRIPTION

Chemically, Antivert® (meclizine HCl) is 1-(p-chloro-α-phe-nylbenzyl) -4- (m -methylbenzyl) piperazine dihydrochloride monohydrate.

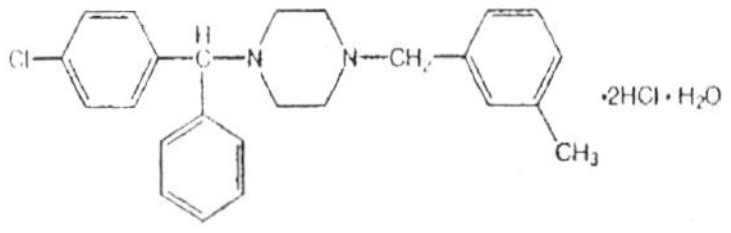

Inert ingredients for the tablets are: dibasic calcium phos-phate; magnesium stearate; polyethylene glycol; starch; su-crose. The 12.5 mg tablets also contain: Blue 1. The 25 mg tablets also contain: Yellow 6 Lake; Yellow 10 Lake. The 50 mg tablets also contain: Blue 1 Lake; Yellow 10 Lake.

ACTIONS

Antivert is an antihistamine which shows marked protec-tive activity against nebulized histamine and lethal doses of intravenously injected histamine in guinea pigs. It has a marked effect in blocking the vasodepressor response to his-tamine, but only a slight blocking action against acetylcho-line. Its activity is relatively weak in inhibiting the spasmo-genic action of histamine on isolated guinea pig ileum.

INDICATIONS

Based on a review of this drug by the National Academy of Sciences-National Research Council and/or other in-formation, FDA has classified the indications as follows:
Effective: Management of nausea and vomiting, and diz-ziness associated with motion sickness.
Possibly Effective: Management of vertigo associated with diseases affecting the vestibular system.
Final classification of the less than effective indications requires further investigation.

CONTRAINDICATIONS

Meclizine HCl is contraindicated in individuals who have shown a previous hypersensitivity to it.

WARNINGS

Since drowsiness may, on occasion, occur with use of this drug, patients should be warned of this possibility and cau-tioned against driving a car or operating dangerous machinery.
Patients should avoid alcoholic beverages while taking this drug. Due to its potential anticholinergic action, this drug should be used with caution in patients with asthma, glau-coma, or enlargement of the prostate gland.

USAGE IN CHILDREN
Clinical studies establishing safety and effectiveness in chil-dren have not been done; therefore, usage is not recom-mended in children under 12 years of age.
USAGE IN PREGNANCY
Pregnancy Category B. Reproduction studies in rats have shown cleft palates at 25–50 times the human dose. Epide-miological studies in pregnant women, however, do not in-dicate that meclizine increases the risk of abnormalities when administered during pregnancy. Despite the animal findings, it would appear that the possibility of fetal harm is remote. Nevertheless, meclizine, or any other medication, should be used during pregnancy only if clearly necessary.

ADVERSE REACTIONS

Drowsiness, dry mouth and, on rare occasions, blurred vi-sion have been reported.

DOSAGE AND ADMINISTRATION

Vertigo:
For the control of vertigo associated with diseases affecting the vestibular system, the recommended dose is 25 to 100 mg daily, in divided dosage, depending upon clinical re-sponse.
Motion Sickness:
The initial dose of 25 to 50 mg of Antivert should be taken one hour prior to embarkation for protection against motion sickness. Thereafter, the dose may be repeated every 24 hours for the duration of the journey.

HOW SUPPLIED

Antivert®—12.5 mg tablets:
Bottles of 100 (NDC 0662-2100-66), (NDC 0049-2100-66)
Bottles of 1000 (NDC 0662-2100-82), (NDC 0049-2100-82)
Antivert®/25—25 mg tablets:
Bottles of 100 (NDC 0662-2110-66), (NDC 0049-2110-66)
Bottles of 1000 (NDC 0662-2110-82), (NDC 0049-2110-82)
Antivert®/50—50 mg tablets:
Bottles of 100 (NDC 0662-2140-66), (NDC 0049-2140-66)
Revised June 1996   69-2148-00-8

Figure 1–1. Antivert tablets. (Reprinted with permission from *Physicians' Desk Reference,* 2001, p. 2469.)

effects. Molloy (1987) reported on an older woman with memory impairment, confusion, disorientation, paranoia, and loss of independence. These symptoms decreased following cessation, after several years of use of meclizine, and then promptly returned on reuse of meclizine.

Manning, Scandale, Manning, and Gengo (1992) explored the CNS effects of meclizine and dimenhydrate (Dramamine). Their results "demonstrate that both dimenhydrinate and meclizine, in recommended doses, produce drowsiness and impaired mental performance greater than a placebo." These authors attempt to "interpret the meaning of the observed decrement in test scores" by comparing their results to the effects of ethanol: "Ethanol serves as a unique drug to reference degree of impairment because there are epidemiologic data that relate to blood alcohol concentrations with a known risk (0.07%) for being involved in a traffic accident." A comparison of the data demonstrates that the effect of dimenhydrinate and meclizine on mental reaction time is equal to that observed while blood alcohol levels were 0.04 to 0.06%.

Kennedy, Wood, Graybiel, and McDonough (1966) performed psychomotor tests and questionnaires on healthy young adults after administering therapeutic doses of several different medications used for motion sickness, including meclizine, and hyoscine (scopolamine). Their results showed no significant decrease in several psychomotor tests, but they did find that meclizine had a significant detrimental effect on balance tests that involved standing on a balance beam. A possible caveat to this study is the fact that the tests were performed within 1 to 2 hours of drug ingestion, whereas later studies (Manning et al., 1992) showed that meclizine had its peak CNS effect 9 hours after dosing.

Lauter, Lynch, Wood, and Schoeffler (1999) performed a battery of tests on normal subjects using meclizine and also noted increased subjective drowsiness and decrease in eye–hand reaction test scores. Interestingly, they found that these subjects had improved eye–hand reaction tasks at 2 days after medication compared with placebo. The implications of this are unknown, but the authors suggest that there may be a "cortical activating" effect related to CNS plasticity. In other words, they suspect that the CNS reaction to a CNS sedative would be to overcompensate and create an improvement in reaction time. Contrary to current popular thinking among vestibular specialists, they infer that early short-term use of meclizine may actually enhance vestibular rehabilitation and central compensation.

Behavioral Recommendations

Fifteen percent of the patients in the study by Sloane et al. (1994) received behavioral recommendations. This finding appears to be consistent with previous reports of psychologic and psychiatric factors associated with dizziness. Numerous researchers have noted a correlation between vestibular disorders and anxiety or panic disorder (Jacob, 1996; Sloane, Hartman & Mitchell, 1994). Whether vestibular disorders may lead to panic disorder or whether vestibular complaints are consequential of panic disorder is a subject of much speculation and research.

Alvord (1991) noted that "dizzy" patients scheduled for ENG had a much higher self-assessment of anxiety than did their non-dizzy patients scheduled for auditory-evoked potential tests or subjects with no medical complaints. Hoffman, O'Leary, and Munjack (1994) reported abnormal scores on the vestibular autorotation test on all patients seen in a panic disorder clinic. These patients were not selected or excluded based on a complaint of dizziness. Jacob (1988) offers a historical perspective on the subject and proposes possible theories as to the cause and effect relationship of panic disorder and the vestibular system: Vestibular evaluations were performed on 21 patients with a history of panic disorder or agoraphobia. He found a high (71 to 75%) incidence of abnormal caloric and posturography scores in these patients. Sklare, Stein, Pikus, and Uhde

(1990) also report that 71% of patients with a history of panic disorder had some abnormality on ENG testing.

It is interesting that *The Anxiety and Phobia Workbook* (Bourne, 1995) includes the following quote: "It is common for the agoraphobic to avoid a variety of situations. Some of these include: (1) Crowded public places such as grocery stores, department stores, restaurants, (2) Enclosed or confined places such as tunnels, bridges, or the hairdresser's chair, (3) Public transportation such as trains, subways, planes, (4) Being home alone." Many of these situations sound strikingly familiar to the complaints of patients with vestibular loss, particularly "fear of crowded spaces (moving visual fields?), tunnels (optokinetic effect?), and the hairdressers chair (BPPV?)." It seems possible that some patients diagnosed with panic and anxiety disorder may have an undiagnosed contributing vestibular disorder. Currently, this is pure speculation, and structured clinical studies would be required before any conclusions can be drawn.

Hyperventilation

Hyperventilation is an anxiety disorder rather than a vestibular disorder, but many patients who experience hyperventilation have as their primary complaints dizziness and lightheadedness that they feel is unprovoked. Many patients suffering from dizziness associated with hyperventilation syndrome are unaware of any coexisting symptoms until they are questioned by a clinician. Drachman and Hart (1972) reported that hyperventilation contributed to complaints of dizziness in 25 of 104 patients evaluated and was the sole cause in four patients. Sama, Meikle, and Jones (1995) reported similar results, stating that hyperventilation caused dizziness in 5% of subjects and was a contributing factor in another 21%. Pathophysiology of hyperventilation will be discussed in Chapter 3.

Observation and Reassurance

Sloane et al. (1994) report that 71.8% of patients underwent "observation" and 41.6% received "reassurance." The article does not elaborate on the criteria for or the outcome of these management strategies. Some dizzy patients will experience resolution of symptoms without evaluation or treatment. Kroenke et al. (1992) report, however, that more than 70% of patients with an initial complaint of dizziness did not have a resolution of symptoms at 2-week follow-up, and of those patients with persistent dizziness, 63% reported experiencing symptoms over a period longer than 3 months. In a prior study by some of the same authors (Kroenke & Mangelsdorff, 1989), 47% of patients complaining of dizziness had no improvement after 11 months. Yardley et al. (1998) report that 30% of patients reporting dizziness have had symptoms for longer than 5 years. Nazareth et al. (1999) performed an 18-month follow-up on the same group of patients in the Yardley et al. (1998) study and found that "24% were more handicapped and 20% had recurrent dizziness, while 20% had improved." These studies suggest that the complaint of dizziness is often associated with persistent symptoms, and simple observation and reassurance are not appropriate in many cases.

Ongoing Searches for Effective Treatment

A recent Internet survey entitled "Coping with Dizziness" (www.conciliocrea-tive.com) indicates that 66% of respondents report suffering from dizziness for at least 1 year. Dizzy patients tend to be persistent in trying to find effective relief from their symptoms. The same Internet survey reveals that 38% of respondents have seen four or more physicians about their dizziness. These survey respondents, of course, are unlikely to represent a random sample of the population because this survey is offered on a Web site designed to provide information about dizziness. Nonetheless, it appears that a significant number of chronically dizzy patients have difficulty finding HCPs that are able to provide effective treatment.

The Importance of Critical Thinking

Most patients play no active role in their own health care and rely totally on the HCP to make management decisions. Consumers of health care services have an overly optimistic view of the effectiveness of medical treatment and rarely question whether the recommended treatment has proved effective (Domenigh-etti, Grilli, & Liberati, 1998). The onus is therefore on the practicing HCP to be sure that the recommended treatment has undergone rigorous clinical trials and is shown to be an effective treatment for most patients with a given diagnosis.

Evidence-based medicine (EBM) has been a subject of considerable debate in the past several years, with most related publications emanating from England and Canada. EBM has been described as "the conscientious, explicit, and judicious use of current best-evidence in making decisions about the care of individual patients. The practice of [EBM] means integrating individual clinical expertise with the best available external clinical evidence from systematic research" (Sackett, Richardson, Rosenberg, & Haynes, 1996). Historically, some well-established medical practices have proved ineffective or even harmful when subjected to rigorous clinical trials. For example, as recently as 1970, antiar-rhythmic medications were prescribed for patients with asymptomatic ventri-cular arrhythmia. After clinical studies were completed, it was learned that death rates actually increased with use of these drugs, and this practice has been discontinued (Braunwald & Antman, 1997).

How do these well-established practices become well established? Typically, these practices are based on the evidence or on current clinical thinking at the time the practice is conceived or are proposed by recognized experts and accepted without question. It is the responsibility off *all* HCPs to question the techniques proposed by their predecessors and either support or participate in clinical examination of current practice patterns (Gates, 1999).

The previous review of primary care management of dizziness demonstrates that one of the most frequent treatment recommendations, medication, does not hold up under the criteria of EBM practice. Canalith repositioning procedures and vestibular rehabilitation (discussed in Chapter 6), however, have been proven effective in providing relief from chronic dysequilibrium and motion and position provoked vertigo. Based on recent clinical evidence, the previous apparent equation of "dizziness equals meclizine" must be reconsidered.

Although some causes of dizziness can be definitively diagnosed only by MRI or laboratory tests, these diseases are rare and typically present some clinical signs or symptoms suggestive of "central" pathology. A directed history and brief physical examination often reveal which patients require the tests mentioned previously. Vestibular evaluation, including ENG, has also been shown to be very sensitive to lesions of the cerebellum or brain stem. Vestibular evaluation has been demonstrated to be more cost effective than MRI or laboratory tests in determining the cause of vertigo (Stewart et al., 1999).

Unfortunately, most dizzy patients never see a specialist who is capable of providing comprehensive vestibular evaluation and treatment. The need for increased awareness by both the public and PCPs is clear, as is the need for more vestibular specialists and balance clinics.

References

Alvord, L. S. (1991). Psychological status of patients undergoing electronystagmography. *J Am Acad Audiol*, *2*, 261–265.

Antman, E. M., Lau, J., Kupelnick, B., Mosteller, F., & Chalmers, T. C. (1992). A comparison of results of meta-analyses of randomized control trials and recommendations of clinical experts. Treatments for myocardial infarction. *JAMA*, *268*(2), 240–248.

Bauch, C. D. (1992). Tests of function versus tests of structure. *Am J Audiol*, 17–18.

Bird, J. C., Beynon, G. J., Prevost, A. T., & Bagulry, D. M. (1998). An analysis of referral patterns for dizziness in the primary care setting. *Br J Gen Pract*, *48*, 1828–1832.

Boult, C., Murphy, J., Sloane, P., Mor, V., & Drone, C. (1991). The relation of dizziness to functional decline. *J Am Geriatr Soc*, *39*, 858–861.

Bourne, E. J. (1995). *The anxiety and phobia workbook*. Oakland, CA: New Harbinger.

Brandt, T. (1991). Medical and physical therapy. In Brandt, T. (Ed.), *Vertigo: Its multisensory syndromes* (pp. 15–17). New York: Springer-Verlag.

Braunwald, E., & Antman, E. M. (1997). Evidence-based coronary care. *Ann Intern Med*, *126*, 551–556.

Burke, M. (1995). Dizziness in the elderly: etiology and treatment. *Nurse Pract*, *20*(12), 28–35.

Clark, D. B., Hirsch, B. E., Smith, M. G., Furman, J. M., & Jacob, R. G. (1994). Panic in otolaryngology patients presenting with dizziness or hearing loss. *Am J Psychiatry*, *151*, 1223–1225.

Clark, M. R., Sullivan, M. D., & Katon, W. J. (1993). Psychiatric and medical factors associated with disability in patients with dizziness. *Psychosomatics*, *34*(5), 409–415.

Cohen, B., & deJong, J. M. B. (1972). Meclizine and placebo in treating vertigo of vestibular origin. *Arch Neurol*, *27*(2), 129–135.

Colledge, N., Barr-Hamilton, R. M., Lewis, S. J., Sellar, R. J., & Wilson, J. A. (1996). Evaluations of investigations to diagnose the cause of dizziness in elderly people: a community based controlled study. *BMJ*, *313*, 788–792.

Dahl, E., Offer-Ohlson, D., Lillevoid, P. E., & Sandvik, L. (1984). Transdermal scopolamine, oral meclizine, and placebo in motion sickness. *Clin Pharmacol Ther*, *36*(1), 116–120.

Day, J., Freer, C. E., Dixon, A. K., Coni, N., Hall, L. D., Sims, C., et al. (1990). Magnetic resonance imaging of the brain and brain-stem in elderly patients with dizziness. *Age Ageing*, *19*, 144–150.

Desmond, A. L. (2000). Vestibular rehabilitation. In M. Valente, H. Hosford-Dunn, & R. J. Roeser (Eds.), *Audiology treatment* (pp. 639–667). New York: Theime Medical Publishers.

Desmond, A. L., & Touchette, D. A. (1998). Cost effective management of the dizzy patient. *Micromed Tech*, *21*, 1–7.

Domenighetti, G., Grilli, R., & Liberati, A. (1998). Promoting consumers' demand for evidence-based medicine. *Int J Technol Assess Health Care*, *14*(1), 97–105.

Drachman, D. A., & Hart, C. W. (1972). An approach to the dizzy patient. *Neurology*, *22*, 323–333.

Enloe, L., & Shields, R. (1997). Evaluation of health-related quality of life in individuals with vestibular disease using disease-specific and general outcome measures. *Phys Ther*, *77*(9), 890–903.

Gates, G. (1999). So where's the evidence? *Otolaryngol Head Neck Surg*, *120*(5), 619–620.

Ghali, W., Saits, R., Sargious, P., & Hershman, W. (1999). Evidence-based medicine and the real world: understanding the controversy. *J Eval Clin Pract*, *5*(2), 133–138.

Grimby, A., & Rosenhall, U. (1995). Health related quality of life in old age. *Gerontology*, *41*, 286–298.

Gizzi, M., Riley, E., & Molinari, S. (1996). The diagnostic value of imaging the patient with dizziness. *Arch Neurol*, *53*, 1299–1304.

Hirose, G., & Halmagyi, G. M. (1996). Brain tumors and balance disorders. In Baloh, R. W. & Halmagyi, G. M. (Eds.), *Disorders of the vestibular system* (pp. 446–460). New York: Oxford University Press.

Hoffman, D., O'Leary, D., & Munjack, D. (1994). Autorotation test abnormalities of the horizontal and vertical vestibulo-ocular reflex in panic disorder. *Arch Otolaryngol Head Neck Surg*, *110*, 259–269.

Honrubia, V., Bell, T., Harris, M. R., Baloh, R. W., & Fisher, L. M. (1996). Quantitative evaluation of dizziness characteristics and impact on quality of life. *Am J Otol*, *17*(4), 95–102.

Jacob, R. G. (1988). Panic disorder and the vestibular system. *Psychiatr Clin North Am*, *11*(2), 361–374.

Jacob, R. G. (1996). Psychiatric aspects of vestibular disorders. In Baloh, R. W. & Halmagyi, G. M. (Eds.), *Disorders of the vestibular system* (pp. 509–528). New York: Oxford University Press.

Katsarkas, A. (1994). Dizziness in aging: A retrospective study of 1194 cases. *Otolaryngol Head Neck Surg*, *110*(3), 29–30.

Kennedy, R., Wood, C., Graybiel, A., & McDonough, R. (1966). Side effects of some antimotion sickness drugs as measured by psychomotor test and questionnaires. *Aerospace Med*, *37*(4), 408–411.

Koch, H., & Smith, M. C. (1985). Office based ambulatory care for patients 75 years old and over. *National ambulatory medical care survey, 1980 and 1981*. Advance data from vital and health statistics. No. 110, DHHS Publication Number (PHS) 85-1250. Hyattsville, MD: Public Health Service.

Kroenke, K., Arrington, M. E., & Mangelsdorff, A. D. (1990). The prevalence of symptoms in medical outpatients and the adequacy of therapy. *Arch Intern Med*, *150*, 1685–1689.

Kroenke, K., Hoffman, R., & Einstadter, D. (2000). How common are various causes of dizziness? *South Med J*, *93*(2), 160–167.

Kroenke, K., Lucas, C., Rosenberg, M., Scherokman, B., & Herbers, J. (1994). One-year outcome for patients with a chief complaint of dizziness. *J Gen Intern Med*, *9*, 684–689.

Kroenke, K., Lucas, C., Rosenberg, M., Scherokman, B., Herbers, J., Wehrle, P., et al. (1992). Causes of persistent dizziness: a prospective study of 100 patients in ambulatory care. *Ann Intern Med*, *17*(11), 898–904.

Kroenke, K., & Mangelsdorff, D. (1989). Common symptoms in ambulatory care: incidence, evaluation, therapy, and outcome. *Am J Med*, *86*, 262–266.

Kutscher, A., Zegarelli, E. V., Hyman, G. A., & Tovell, H. M. (1966). A case report: Prolonged use of meclizine hydrochloride with total absence of side effects. *Ann Allergy*, *24*, 246–247.

Lauter, J., Lynch, O., Wood, S., & Schoeffler, L. (1999). Physiological and behavioral effects of an antivertigo antihistamine in adults. *Percept Mot Skills*, *88*, 707–732.

Lawson, J., Fitzgerald, J., Birchall, J., Aldren, C. P., & Kenny, R. A. (1999). Diagnosis of geriatric patients with severe dizziness. *J Am Geriatr Soc*, *47*, 12–17.

Li, J. C., Li, C. J., Epley, J., & Weinberg, L. (2000). Cost-effective management of benign positional vertigo using canalith repositioning. *Otolaryngol Head Neck Surg*, *122*(3), 334–339.

Lord, S., Clark, R., & Webster, I. (1991). Postural stability and associated physiological factors in a population of aged persons. *J Gerontol Med Sci*, *46*(3), M69–M76.

Manning, C., Scandale, L., Manning, E., & Gengo, F. (1992). Central nervous system effects of meclizine and dimenhydrinate: Evidence of acute tolerance to antihistamines. *J Clin Pharmacol*, *32*, 996–1002.

McElmore, T., & Delozier, J. (1985). National ambulatory medical care survey. In National center for health statistics: Advance data from vital and health statistics, DHHS publication No. (PHS) 87-1250. Hyattsville, MD: Government Printing Office, 1987.

Molloy, D. W. (1987). Memory loss, confusion, and disorientation in an elderly woman taking meclizine. *J Am Geriatr Soc*, *35*, 454–456.

Nazareth, I., Yardley, L., Owen, N., & Luxon, L. (1999). Outcome of symptoms of dizziness in a general practice community sample. *Fam Pract*, *16*(6), 616–618.

Newman, C. W., & Jacobson, G. P. (1993). Application of self-report scales in balance function handicap assessment. *Semin Hear*, *14*(4), 363–375.

Ojala, M., Ketonen, L., & Palo, J. (1988). The value of CT and very low field MRI in the etiologic diagnosis of dizziness. *Acta Neurol Scandinavia*, *78*, 26–29.

Physicians, Desk Reference (2000). 55th ed. Montvale, NJ: Medical Economics Company. Retrieved November 3, 2003, from www.PDR.net.

Prass, R. Atlantic Coast Ear Specialists. Retrieved November 3, 2003, from www.earaces.com.

Sackett, D. L., Richardson, W. S., Rosenberg, W., & Haynes, R. B. (1996). Evidence-based medicine: how to practice and teach EBM. *Br J Audiol*, *33*, 17–27.

Saddat, D., O'Leary, D. P., Pulec, J. L., & Kitano, H. (1995). Comparison of vestibular autorotation and caloric testing. *Otolaryngol Head Neck Surg*, *113*(3), 215–222.

Sama, A., Meikle, J. C. E., & Jones, N. S. (1995). Hyperventilation and dizziness: Case reports and management. *Br J Gen Pract*, *49*(2), 79–82.

Shapiro, D. (1999). Geriatric demographics and the practice of otolaryngology. *Ear Nose Throat J*, *78*(6), 418–421.

Shepard, N.T., Telian, S. A., & Smith-Wheelock, M. (1990). Habituation and balance retraining therapy: A retrospective review. *Neurol Clin*, *8*(2), 459–475.

Shepard, N. T., Telian, S. A., & Smith-Wheelock, M. (1996). *Practical management of the balance disorder patient*. San Diego: Singular Publishing Group.

Sklare, D. A., Stein, M. B., Pikus, A. M., & Uhde, T. W. (1990). Dysequilibrium and audiovestibular function in panic disorder: Symptom profiles and test findings. *Am J Otol*, *11*(5), 338–341.

Sloane, P. D. (1989). Dizziness in primary care: Results from national ambulatory medical care survey. *J Fam Pract*, *29*(1), 33–38.

Sloane, P., Blazer, D., & George, L. (1989). Dizziness in a community elderly population. *J Am Geriatr Soc*, *37*(2), 101–108.

Sloane, P. D., & Dallara, J. (1999). Clininical research and geriatric dizziness: the blind men and the elephant. *J Am Geriatr Soc*, *47*(1), 113–114.

Sloane, P. D., Dallara, J., Roach, C., Bailey, K. E., Mitchell, M., & McNutt, R. (1994). Management of dizziness in primary care. *J Am Board Fam Pract*, *7*, 1–8.

Sloane, P. D., Hartman, M., & Mitchell, C. M. (1994). Psychological factors associated with chronic dizziness in patients aged 60 and over. *J Am Geriatr Soc*, *42*, 847–853.

Smith, D. B. (1990). Dizziness: A clinical perspective. *Neurol Clin*, *8*(2), 2612–2617.

Stewart, M., Chen, A. Y., Wyatt, J. R., Favrot, S., Beinart, S., Coker, N. J., et al. (1999). Cost-effectiveness of the diagnostic evaluation of vertigo. *Laryngoscope*, *109*, 600–605.

Sullivan, M., Clark, M. R., Katon, W. J., Fischl, M., Russo, J., Dobie, R.A., et al. (1993). Psychiatric and otologic diagnoses in patients complaining of dizziness. *Arch Intern Med*, *153*, 1479–1484.

Tinetti, M., Williams, C., & Gill, T. (2000). Dizziness among older adults: a possible geriatric syndrome. *Ann Intern Med*, *132*(5), 337–344.

United States Census Bureau. (February 8, 1999). Statistical brief. *Sixty-five plus in the United States*. Retrieved November 3, 2003, from www.census.gov/socdemo.

Ware, J., Phillips, J., Benson, B., & Adamczyk, J. (1996). Assessment tools: functional health status and patient satisfaction. *Am J Med Qual*, *11*(1), S50–S53.

Yardley, L., Owen, N., Nazareth, I., & Luxon, L. (1998). Prevalence and presentation of dizziness in a general practice community sample of working age people. *Br J Gen Prac*, *48*, 1131–1135.

Zee, D. (1985). Perspectives on the pharmocotherapy of vertigo. *Arch Otolaryngol*, *111*, 609–612.

2

Function and Dysfunction of the Vestibular System

Normal Function of the Vestibular System

The primary role of the balance system is to allow humans to interact and maintain contact with their surroundings in a safe, efficient manner. As humans move through their environment, information is gathered through their visual, somatosensory, and vestibular senses and sent to the brain stem for integration and finally to the cortex for perception and processing (Fig. 2–1). The visual and somatosensory reference information is constantly changing as a function of movement, but the vestibular reference— gravity— is unchanging. As long as the information arriving from these three sources is predictable and nonconflicting, equilibrium is maintained and there is little thought regarding balance.

When a sensory conflict occurs, the brain must efficiently and quickly (reflexively) adjust the level of priority given to the conflicting incoming information, or a sensation of imbalance may occur. Because the known constant in the mix is gravity, humans tend to rely more on vestibular information for maintenance of dynamic balance than they do on proprioceptive or visual information (when the peripheral vestibular system is damaged, this may change).

Allum and Pfaltz (1985) hypothesized that vestibular information contributes 65% to dynamic body stability; vision and proprioception provide less of a contribution. Standing balance, however, does not rely primarily on vestibular information. Colledge et al. (1994) and Hobeika (1999) report that proprioception is the major contributor to standing balance; however, when proprioceptive input is not helpful (i.e., moving or compliant surface), vision becomes the primary source of information.

In summary, the balance system is dynamic and quickly responds to changes in visual, vestibular, and proprioceptive feedback. Although the peripheral vestibular system is most often of primary importance, the interactions between the peripheral vestibular inputs, vision, and proprioception in the brain are crucial to the maintenance of balance.

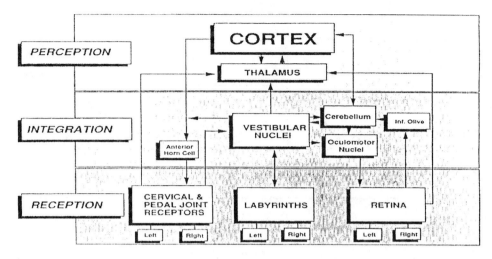

Figure 2–1. Vestibular reception, integration, and perception: The neuroanatomy of dizziness depicting the primary structures involved in the perception of balance and equilibrium organized as a hierarchy. Corollary and redundant information from peripheral receptors converges at central integration sites or projects directly to thalamic relay nuclei and cortex. Some efferent and reflex control mechanisms are depicted. [Reprinted with permission from Brown, J. J. (1993). A system oriented approach to the dizzy patient. In: I. K. Aranberg (Ed.), *Dizziness and balance disorders* (pp. 11–24). New York: Kugler Publications].

Peripheral Vestibular Anatomy

The peripheral vestibular apparatus consists of matched pairs of sensors that are stimulated by any type of movement; specific sensors are responsible for specific movements. These sensors are located within the labyrinth, which is a series of interconnected canals and cavities located within the petrous portion of the temporal bone (Fig. 2–2). The outer wall of the labyrinth is known as the *bony labyrinth,* which is filled with perilymphatic fluid. Perilymphatic fluid has a similar chemical composition to cerebrospinal fluid and has a high sodium (Na) to potassium (K) ratio.

Inside the bony labyrinth and suspended in perilymphatic fluid lies the membranous labyrinth. The fluid inside the membranous labyrinth is known as *endolymphatic fluid,* and it has a chemical composition that contrasts with the perilymph on the other side of the membrane. Endolymph has a high ratio of potassium to sodium. All five sensory organs are housed within the membranous labyrinth. The five sensors are commonly known as the utricle, the saccule, and the three cristae ampullaris, one each in each of the three semicircular canals. The utricle and saccule are known as the *otolith structures.* The utricle plays a large role in postural control and primarily senses changes in orientation to gravity and horizontal movements, such as moving forward in a car. It is located within the vestibule, which has open fluid (endolymph) communication with the semicircular canals. The utricle has been described as a "membranous tube" (Wright & Schwade, 2000) that is primarily made up of otoconial membrane,

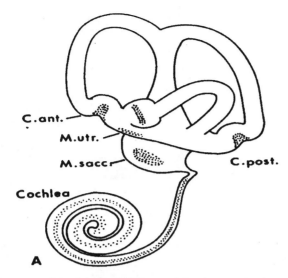

Figure 2–2. Schematic of the labyrinth. The semicircular canals sit at right angles to each other so that any tilt of the head will stimulate endolymph movement in at least one canal. C. ant, cupula of the anterior canal; C. post., cupula of the posterior canal; M. utr, macula of the utricle; M. sacc, macula of the saccule. (Reprinted and adapted with permission from Leigh, R. J., & Zee, D. S. (1991). *The neurology of eye movements* (2nd ed.) Philadelphia: F.A. Davis.)

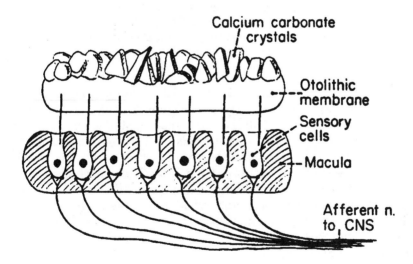

Figure 2–3. Graphic illustration of an otolith organ with sensory cells projecting into the gelatinous otolithic membrane. Otoconia (calcium carbonate crystals) are situated on the otolithic membrane. (Reprinted and adapted with permission from Baloh, R.W. & Honrubia, V. (1990). *Clinical neurophysiology of the vestibular system.* Philadelphia: F.A. Davis.)

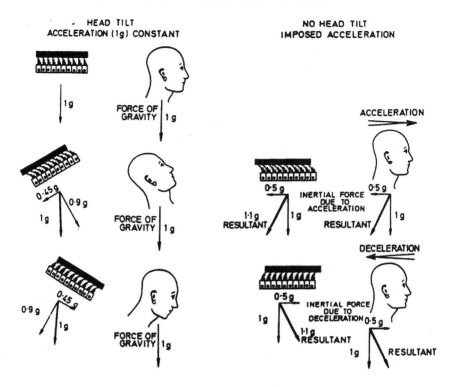

Figure 2–4. Utricular organ showing how the sensory cells are stimulated by displacement of the otoconial membrane (solid black) when the head is tilted and when undergoing fore to aft acceleration. Note that acceleration is similar to backward tilt. Deceleration is similar to forward tilt. (Reprinted with permission from Gresty, M. A. (1996). Vestibular tests in evolution. I. Otolith testing. In: R. W. Baloh, & G. M. Halmagyi (Eds.), *Disorders of the vestibular system* (pp. 243–255). New York: Oxford University Press.)

sensory cells, and supporting structures (Fig. 2–3). The otoconial membrane (also known as the macula) consists of a layer of calcium carbonate crystals known as *otoconia.* Just below the otoconia lies a gelatinous membrane through which the sensory cells (hair cells) project. Any movement of the otoconia relative to the supporting structure results in stimulation of the sensory cells. The otoconia are small grain- or rice-shaped particles with a density that is much greater than the surrounding endolymph. It is this difference in density that allows the utricle to respond transiently to linear acceleration and in a more protracted fashion to head tilt. With a sudden forward movement, the supporting structures will move synchronously with the head (Fig. 2–4). The density (and therefore the weight) of the otoconia cause them to lag behind head movement. After several seconds of linear forward movement (such as accelerating in a car), the otoconia "catch up," and the utricular response is exhausted. A tilt of the head causes a prolonged response from the utricle. Because of the increased density of the otoconia, they are sensitive to gravity. When the head is tilted, the weight of the otoconia cause them to shift in relation to the supporting structures, again resulting in stimulation of the underlying sensory cells. Unlike the transient response noted

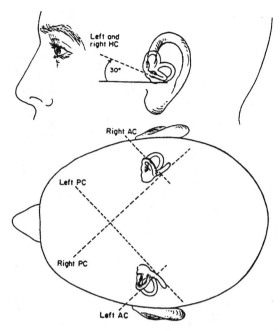

Figure 2–5. Orientation of the semicircular canals within the head. HC, horizontal canal; PC, posterior canal; AC, anterior canal. (Reprinted and adapted with permission from Baloh, R. W. & Honrubia, V. (1990). *Clinical neurophysiology of the vestibular system.* Philadelphia: F.A. Davis.)

for linear movements, the sensory cells will continue to respond as long as the head remains in the same position. It is for this reason that the utricle is believed to be the primary sensor for our orientation to gravity and plays such an important role in postural stability.

The saccule is similar in organizational structure to the utricle, but it is oriented in the vertical plane. The saccule lies adjacent to the basal end of the cochlea in an area known as the *spherical recess*. The saccule does not have open fluid communication with the utricle or the semicircular canals; rather, it is connected through the vestibular aqueduct (Wright and Schwade, 2000). The role of the saccule is controversial but is believed primarily to register vertical movements, such as the sensation experienced when moving in an elevator. The role of the saccule in postural control is unclear. At this time, accurate assessment of otolith abnormalities is experimental and not widely accepted (Halmagyi, Colematch, & Curthoys, 1994).

The semicircular canals are responsible for detecting angular head movement in the *pitch* (shaking your head "yes") plane, the *yaw* (shaking your head "no") plane, and the *roll* (tilting your head to the side) plane. The arrangement of the semicircular canals at right angles to each other (Fig. 2–5) causes the inner ear fluid (endolymph) to flow toward or away from the ampulla in at least one canal on each side with any of the above-mentioned head movements. As long as the response registered in each of the matched canals on either side of the head is the same, balance and orientation are maintained. The horizontal canal on one side is

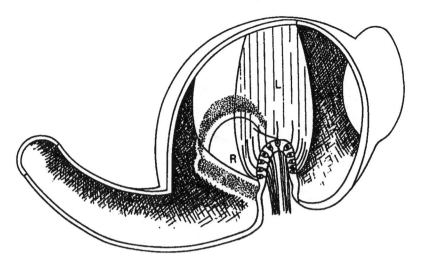

Figure 2–6. Schematic diagram of the sensory structures inside the ampulla of a semicircular duct. The crista (R), which extends across the ampulla, is covered in sensory epithelium. The cilia (hair cells) of the sensory cells project into the cupula (L), a gelatinous mass that fills the space between the surface of the cristae and the opposite wall of the ampulla. (Reprinted and adapted with permission from Wright, C. G., & Schwade, N. D. (2000). Anatomy and physiology of the vestibular system. In: R. J. Roeser, M. Valente, & H. Hossford-Dunn (Eds.), *Audiology diagnosis*. New York: Thieme Medical Publishers.)

matched to the opposite horizontal canal; the posterior canal is matched to the opposite anterior canal (Fig. 2–5). The sensory cells within the semicircular canals (cristae ampullaris) are housed within the ampulla, which is a widening of the bony and membranous portion of each canal. Sitting atop the cristae ampullaris is a gelatinous membrane called the cupula (Fig. 2–6), which extends across the ampulla to close off the lumen of the canal. The cupula has been described as a thin sail-like structure or diaphragm that is exquisitely sensitive to motion. The cupula, unlike the macula of the otoliths, has a density that is similar to the surrounding endolymph and is therefore not sensitive to prolonged static tilt.

Vestibular Hair Cells

The effects of motion and gravity result in stimulation of the vestibular sensory cells. The sensory cells consist of hair cells that (much like the cochlear hair cells) respond to fluid motion. In the case of cochlear hair cells, the stimulation is brought on by sound waves. The vestibular hair cells are stimulated by movement and a position relative to gravity. Each vestibular hair cell has one kinocilium and several stereocilia that are arranged in a "stair-step" pattern. The single kinocilium is the longest of the cilia, and the stereocilia become progressively shorter across the hair cell. In their resting state, each hair cell has a resting electrical potential. With any motion, this potential will change from baseline and may either increase or decrease, depending on hair cell orientation. The structure and arrangement of the cilia allow for the detection of direction of

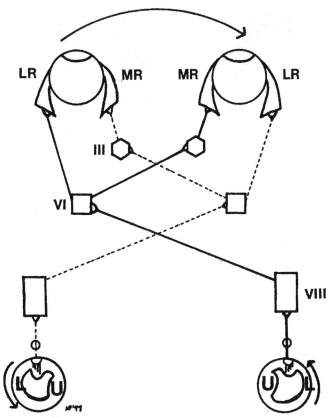

Figure 2–7. Simplified schematic drawing illustrating the basic neurocircuits that mediate the horizontal vestibular ocular reflex. The circular figures at the bottom of the diagram represent the right and left vestibular labyrinth, with "L" indicating the lateral semicircular duct and "U" indicating the utricle. From the cristae of the lateral ducts, neural impulses are relayed through the vestibular nerve to the vestibular nuclei (VIII) and then to the nuclei of the abducens (VI) and oculomotor (III) nerves controlling the medial rectus (MR) and lateral rectus (LR) muscles that move the eyes in the horizontal plane. These pathways involve relatively few neurons so that the stimulus to response time (latency) of the vestibular ocular reflex (VOR) is short. When the head undergoes angular acceleration to the right (large arrow on top), fluid displacement in the lateral duct deflects the stereocilia of the right crista toward the utricle and those of the left crista away from the utricle as indicated by the small arrows. This results in increased neural discharge in the pathway drawn in solid lines and decreased activity in the pathway shown in dotted lines, producing a leftward shift of the eyes because of contraction of the medial and lateral rectus muscles on the left side of each eye. Thus rotation of the head in one direction results in movement of the eyes in the opposite direction. (Reprinted and adapted with permission from Wright, C. G., & Schwade, N. D. (2000). Anatomy and physiology of the vestibular system. In: R. J. Roeser, M. Valente, & H. Hossford-Dunn (Eds.), *Audiology diagnosis*. New York: Thieme Medical Publishers.)

movement. Any movement that causes the stereocilia to flow *toward* the kinocilium results in depolarization and an *increase* in electrical potential, whereas movement that causes the stereocilia to flow *away* from the kinocilium

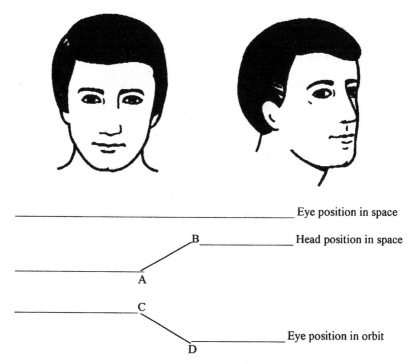

Eye position in space

Head position in space

Eye position in orbit

Figure 2–8. Vestibular ocular reflex (VOR): The role of the VOR is to maintain eye position in space as the head moves. (A) Onset of head movement. (C) Onset of reflexive eye movement in the orbit (typically less than 16 ms after A). This minimal duration of retinal slip accounts for maintenance of gaze stability with head movement. (B, D) A 30-degree excursion of head movement and eye movement in opposite directions demonstrating a gain of one, and in effect visually canceling out the effect of head movement. (Reprinted with permission from Leigh, R. J., & Zee, D. S. (1999). *Neurology of Eye Movements*, New York: Oxford, Fig. 2-4A, p. 30.)

results in hyperpolarization and a *decrease* in electrical potential. An increase in potential is described as *excitatory*, and a decrease in potential is described as *inhibitory*.

In the semicircular canals, the orientation of the hair cells varies. In the horizontal canal, the orientation is such that a purely horizontal head movement to the right would result in endolymph flow toward the ampulla of the right horizontal canal and away from the ampulla of the left horizontal canal. This causes the stereocilia to flow toward the kinocilium on the ipsilateral side (right) and away from the kinocilium on the contralateral side (left). For example, a rightward horizontal head movement will result in an excitatory response from the right labyrinth and a corresponding inhibitory response on the left labyrinth (Fig. 2–7). The hair cell orientation in the anterior and posterior canals is just the opposite. Endolymph flow toward the ampulla in the anterior and posterior canals causes the stereocilia to flow away from the kinocilium and results in an inhibitory response.

Each otolith structure (utricle and saccule) exhibits hair cell orientation in more than one direction. For example, some hair cells are oriented to provide an excitatory response to forward movement, whereas others are oppositely oriented and will result in an inhibitory response. It is believed that the otoliths also work as matched pairs, and any movement causing a primarily excitatory response on one side would be paired against a primarily inhibitory response on the opposite side.

Vestibular Ocular Reflex

The *vestibular ocular reflex (VOR)* can be defined as reflexive eye movement in response to head movement. This short latency response occurs as a direct result of changes in labyrinthine electrical potentials. As in the previous example of a horizontal head movement to the right, the difference in polarization results in asymmetric activity at the level of the vestibular nuclei, with increased activity on the right and a corresponding decrease on the left. The two vestibular nuclei pass this asymmetry along to the ocular motor nuclei, which results in a contraction of the lateral rectus muscle of the left eye and the medial rectus muscle of the right eye. The rectus muscles (which along with the oblique muscles are known as *extraocular muscles*) work in an antagonistic fashion described as the *law of reciprocal innervation.* When there is a contraction of the lateral rectus muscle, there is an equivalent relaxation of the opposing medial rectus muscle (Leigh & Zee, 1991). This response from the extraocular muscles results in eye movement that is equal and opposite to head movement with minimal latency, in effect visually canceling out head movement.

The role of the VOR is to allow for stable gaze (focused clear vision) while the head is moving (Fig. 2–8). Visual acuity degrades when the visual scene moves past the retina at speeds greater than 3 to 5 degrees per second (Leigh & Zee, 1991). A simple demonstration of the VOR can be accomplished while reading this page. Simply hold this page 18 inches in front of you and move your head back and forth at the maximum speed that still allows for clarity and easy reading. Then, with your head stationary, move the page back and forth in front of you at a speed nearly equal to the speed at which you moved your head. A noticeable degradation in visual acuity occurs. It is impossible to move the eyes voluntarily at speeds needed to maintain visual acuity during typical head movements. The latency of response for the VOR is less than 16 milliseconds (ms), whereas the latency for a voluntary eye movement is approximately 70 ms under ideal, predictable conditions. It is much slower (around 200 ms) for unpredictable targets (Leigh & Zee, 1991). The VOR is compromised with damage to one or both peripheral vestibular apparatuses.

Nystagmus and the Vestibular Ocular Reflex

Nystagmus is involuntary rhythmic eye movement that is most often associated with acute labyrinthine pathology or neurologic disease. There is usually a fast and slow phase to nystagmus in which the eye moves slowly in one direction and then makes a rapid jerking motion in the opposite direction. The slow phase of nystagmus is more pertinent toward interpreting pathology, whereas the fast phase is more easily observed.

Conditions causing nystagmus can be elicited either by pathological conditions [vestibular neuritis, Meniere's disease, benign paroxysmal positional vertigo (BPPV), migraine] or by abnormal or excessive stimulation of the labyrinth (caloric or rotational stimulation). Nystagmus does not normally occur during typical head movements. Conditions such as vestibular neuritis and cool caloric irrigation cause a sudden reduction in the output from the affected or stimulated labyrinth. Conditions such as active Meniere's disease, BPPV, and warm caloric irrigation cause a sudden increase in the affected or stimulated labyrinth. Anytime a difference is noted, a sense of rotation occurs, and the eyes deviate away from the stronger side toward the weaker side, causing the slow phase of nystagmus. Viscoelastic forces from elastic connective tissue around the eyes are responsible for the fast phase of nystagmus, which brings the eye back to center (Carl, 1993). These two forces create the rapid jerking motion seen in peripherally generated nystagmus. Nystagmus is usually temporary and ceases when either the asymmetry is resolved, as in BPPV or Meniere's disease, or after sufficient central compensation takes place as in vestibular neuritis.

Normal Eye and Head Speed

It is estimated that the frequency range of head movement encountered in real life is from 0.5 to 5 Hz, and the VOR normally responds efficiently up to frequencies approaching 8 Hz (Gresty, Hess, & Leech, 1977; Sawyer et al., 1994). A variety of voluntary cerebellar modulated eye movements may allow for gaze stability at frequencies below 1 Hz, but only the VOR can allow for gaze stability and clear vision to head movements greater than 2 Hz. For the purposes of this text, head movements that can be measured with a rotary chair (typically below 1 Hz) are considered *low frequency.* Faster head movements (1 to 2 Hz and above) are considered *high frequency.*

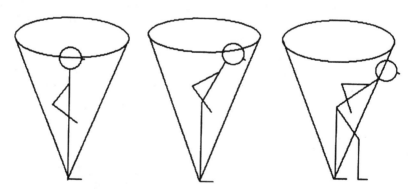

Figure 2–9. Limits of stability (LOS) describes the amount a patient can sway or lean from the center of gravity before falling or before requiring a corrective action. The LOS varies and is affected by height, leg strength, and posture. A patient who exceeds the limit of stability must make a corrective measure to avoid falling.

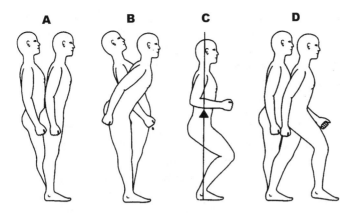

Figure 2–10. Reflexive postural control strategies: (A) Ankle strategy: This is effective for small, slow perturbation near the center of gravity (COG) and results from contraction of the leg muscles while keeping the body aligned with the hips and knees. (B) Hip strategy: This involves movement of the head and hips in opposite directions to counteract weight shift from the COG. (C) Suspensory strategy: This effectively lowers the COG making maintenance of balance easier. (D) Stepping strategy: When the LOS has been exceeded, a stepping motion reestablishes a new COG. (Reprinted with permission from Allison, L. (1995). Balance disorders. In: D. A. Umphred & Mosby (Eds.), *Neurologic rehabilitation* (pp. 802–837). St. Louis: Mosby-Yearbook Inc.

Physiology of the Vestibular Ocular Reflex

It is estimated that human peripheral vestibular afferent fibers have resting potentials of up to 100 spikes per second. Considering that there are about 18,000 vestibular afferents in each labyrinth, the resting activity (or resting potential) received by each vestibular nucleus may be more than one million spikes per second (Curthoys & Halmagyi, 1996). Any head movement results in a change in this resting potential of the peripheral vestibular labyrinths and the vestibular nuclei receive asymmetric inputs from the two vestibular labyrinths. Earlier reports of vestibular physiology described a simple "push–pull" arrangement in which a head movement would cause an excitatory response in one vestibular nucleus and a corresponding, but not necessarily equal, inhibitory response in the contralateral vestibular nucleus. Although this accurately describes the output of the labyrinths, it is now believed that for each head movement, both inhibitory and excitatory responses occur in both vestibular nuclei and that the inhibitory responses are the result of inhibitory commissural connections from the contralateral vestibular nucleus (Curthoys & Halmagyi, 1996). These commissural connections help to explain the process of tonic rebalancing (discussed later in this chapter).

Vestibulospinal Reflex

The vestibulospinal reflex (VSR) helps to maintain and regain postural stability during movement. Much like eye movements, postural adjustments can be either volitional or reflexive. *Volitional postural control* involves the conscious shifting of weight from the center of gravity to achieve an objective such as taking a step or reaching for an object (Allison, 1995). Through the process of motor learning, these types of movements are modified if unsuccessful (such as falling) and refined until individuals understand their limits of stability (LOS) and can move safely in their environment (Fig. 2–9).

Reflexive postural control is associated with the VSR and is a short-latency response to perturbation. There are four known types of reflexive postural adjustment to avoid exceeding the LOS and falling (Fig. 2–10). Ankle strategy results from contraction of the leg muscles to keep the body aligned with the hips and knees. Ankle strategy is appropriate for small, slow perturbation. Hip strategy involves movement of the head and hips to counteract weight shifts away from the center of gravity. Suspensory strategy involves lowering the center of gravity, thereby increasing stability. Stepping strategy is used when other attempts to maintain the center of gravity fail and a new center of gravity must be established.

Dysfunction of the Vestibular System

Static Symptoms

The tonic or resting state of the paired vestibular labyrinths is a delicate balance that can be disrupted by a sudden injury to one or both labyrinths. Conditions responsible for unilateral vestibular injury include vestibular neuritis, Meniere's disease, labyrinthitis (see Common Disorders in this chapter), or surgical procedures such as eighth nerve section or labyrinthectomy (Bohmer, 1996).[1]

Sudden Vestibular Asymmetry

Following a sudden loss or reduction in the function of one labyrinth, a predictable set of clinical signs and symptoms occurs. These "static" symptoms include spontaneous nystagmus, a subjective sensation of vertigo with nausea, postural instability, ataxia, and ocular tilt reaction (OTR) (Curthoys & Halmagyi, 1996; Halmagyi, Gresty, & Gibson, 1979; Leigh & Zee, 1991; Robinson, Zee, Hain, Holmes, & Rosenbug, 1984). These symptoms result from a sudden profound asymmetry in resting activity between the two vestibular nuclei. Whenever there is an imbalance in the output of the vestibular nuclei, a sense of rotation toward the side with the higher resting potential is perceived.

Alexander's law refers to the pattern of nystagmus typically seen during the acute phase (first 1 to 3 days) of peripheral vestibular asymmetry. In Alexander's law, the intensity of nystagmus increases when gaze (to look or stare intently in one direction) is directed toward the fast phase of nystagmus (away from the lesioned side) and decreases when gaze is directed toward the slow phase (toward the lesioned side). OTR indicates tonic imbalance of the activity of the VOR and consists of skew deviation (vertical misalignment), ocular counter-

---

[1]BPPV causes transient vestibular asymmetry and does not require an alteration in central processing because the labyrinth itself is restored to homeostasis (the state of dynamic equilibrium of the internal environment of the body).

rolling (fixed torsion) of the eyes, and head tilt toward the side with a lesion. The reader is referred to Leigh and Zee (1991) for a complete review.

Tonic Rebalancing

Over a period of hours to days, the symptoms of vertigo and nausea, as well as nystagmus, diminish considerably through the process of vestibular adaptation. Because evidence suggests that labyrinthine receptors and peripheral neurons do not regenerate, the process of adaptation is thought to be a result of a variety of possible mechanisms within the central nervous system (CNS) (Curthoys & Halmagyi, 1996). The precise mechanism is not fully understood, but most researchers believe that the process of vestibular adaptation is a function of alterations in activity of the vestibular nuclei. Smith and Curthoys (1989) and Curthoys and Halmagyi (1996) offer thorough reviews of studies pertaining to "tonic rebalancing" following unilateral labyrinthine loss.

Loss of Contralateral Inhibitory Influence

Following the sudden loss or reduction in function of one labyrinth, there is an immediate dramatic *decrease* in the resting activity of the ipsilateral vestibular nucleus. There is also an immediate *increase* in resting activity in the contralateral vestibular nucleus, which is likely the result of the loss of inhibitory commissural connections normally received from the lesioned side (Igarashi, 1984; Smith & Curthoys, 1989). Simply stated, the two vestibular nuclei are interactive and dependent on each other to maintain equal resting outputs. Each vestibular nucleus exerts some inhibitory influence on the other. When the function of one vestibular nucleus is lost, the other vestibular nucleus temporarily responds with an increase in activity over and above its normal resting level of activity. This creates a sudden profound asymmetry in the two vestibular nuclei and leads to the above-mentioned signs and symptoms of sudden unilateral vestibular deafferentation (UVD).

Cerebellar Clamp

The CNS responds by reducing the resting level of the intact side (a process known as *cerebellar clamp*) and gradually restores activity in the vestibular nucleus on the lesioned side. This process leads to tonic rebalancing and a reduction in static symptoms. Restoration of activity in the vestibular nucleus on the lesioned side should not be confused with restoration of response from the lesioned peripheral labyrinth. This process of tonic rebalancing and the time course for reduction of static symptoms such as spontaneous nystagmus and ocular tilt do not appear to be dependent on visual or physical exercise stimulation (Zee, 1994).

Bechterew's Phenomenon

The rebalancing of neural activity between the two vestibular nuclei becomes evident when a patient suffering previous unilateral vestibular loss, after a period of adaptation, suffers a loss in the contralateral labyrinth. Because the symptoms of sudden unilateral vestibular loss as described previously are believed to result from sudden asymmetry in the resting potentials of the vestibular nuclei, common sense dictates that a loss of function in the remaining labyrinth would result in the absence of, but symmetrical output from, the two vestibular labyrinths. In such a case, however, the patient responds behaviorally as if loss of the remaining labyrinth results in a sudden asymmetry with the well-known pattern of static symptoms of acute unilateral loss (Precht, Shimazu, & Markham, 1966). This is known as _Bechterew's phenomenon,_ which provides evidence of restoration of activity in the vestibular nucleus on the lesioned side.

Role of Commisural Connections

Bienhold and Flohr (1978) described the role of the commisural connections. To determine the role of these connections in vestibular compensation, these researchers surgically destroyed the commisural connections in the frog at various stages of compensation following unilateral labyrinthectomy. Bienhold and Flohr (1978) noted (1) an immediate return of symptoms of unilateral labyrinthectomy, (2) that the level of symptoms was independent of the time allowed and level of compensation, and (3) that no recompensation could be observed. These findings indicate that without these commisural connections allowing for information from the contralateral labyrinth to be received by the lesioned side vestibular nucleus, vestibular adaptation could not take place. The restoration of activity in the vestibular nucleus of the lesioned side may play an important role in the recovery from static symptoms but does not appear to contribute significantly to the reduction of dynamic symptoms (Smith & Curthoys, 1989).

Dynamic Symptoms

Dynamic symptoms include symptoms that occur as a result of head movement secondary to dysfunction of the VOR. Whereas the static symptoms of acute unilateral vestibular loss are quite predictable and easily identified, dynamic symptoms of VOR dysfunction are more subtle and recovery of VOR function is more dependent on external influences.

Oscillopsia

Symptoms of dynamic VOR dysfunction typically do not include complaints of vertigo but rather of visual blurring with head movement (_oscillopsia_) and visual- and motion-provoked dysequilibrium. Brandt (1991) defines oscillopsia as "apparent movement of the visual scene due to involuntary retinal slip in acquired ocular oscillations or deficient VOR." In this context, "acquired ocular oscillations" would be nystagmus, which should be evident to the examiner. Nystagmus is involuntary eye movement associated with tonic imbalance within the peripheral or central vestibular system. When nystagmus is present, this eye movement may prohibit accurate visual fixation or visual following, leading to oscillopsia without head movement. Patients without nystagmus, but with a "deficient VOR," typically experience oscillopsia only when they are moving. Some patients with confirmed (by calorics) bilateral vestibular loss experience no more than mild dysequilibrium, wheres others complain of blurred vision and "bouncing" of their visual world with any head movement. J.C., a physician treated with vestibulotoxic aminoglycosides, reports (1952) that to be able to read he had to hold his head steady by bracing it through the rails of his bed.[44] Otherwise, his heartbeat and pulse caused too much head movement to allow gaze stability. Patients with oscillopsia tend to be asymptomatic when they are not moving. To varying degrees, head movement causes a decrease in visual acuity, which can be easily documented using a standard Snellen eye chart (Longridge & Mallinson, 1984). This technique is discussed in Chapter 3.

Retinal Slip

The basis for these complaints is termed *retinal slip,* the inability to maintain focused, centered vision (foveal vision) with head movements. Retinal slip occurs when the VOR cannot adequately compensate for head movement and images do not remain stable on the retina. Visual acuity is best when an image is centered and stable on the retina. A gradual decline in visual acuity is noted as visual images move across the retina at increasing speeds. No significant decrease is noted when images move across the retina at speeds of two to three degrees per second, but at four to five degrees per second and above, gaze stability and visual acuity are compromised (Demer, Honrubia, & Baloh, 1994; Leigh & Zee, 1991). *Gaze stability* may be defined as the ability to maintain foveal vision during head movements.

When retinal slip occurs and visual acuity is compromised, a sensory conflict between perceived visual, vestibular, and somatosensory information can occur. Patients with vestibular deficits tend to become more reliant on accurate visual and somatosensory feedback for maintenance of equilibrium, orientation, and balance. In the early stages following vestibular injury, there is a noted greater reliance on visual information (Keshner, 1994). Gaze instability leads to inaccurate visual feedback, affecting appropriate sensory integration of the incoming information.

Recalibrating the Vestibular Ocular Reflex

Recovery of the VOR is believed to occur primarily as a result of CNS and cerebellar plasticity and is possibly part of the process of cerebellar clamp. The retinal slip caused by VOR dysfunction leads to an "error signal" in that images would be blurred during locomotion. CNS plasticity uses this error signal and gradually recalibrates the output (or gain[2]) of the VOR in an effort to enhance stable and clear vision. Several investigators have demonstrated that VOR gain and direction can be modified by subjecting patients with normal vestibular function to error signals (Demer, Porter, Goldberg, Jenkins, & Schmidt, 1989; Gonshor & Melvill-Jones, 1976; Khater, Baker, & Peterson, 1990). It is believed that the error signal induced by VOR dysfunction triggers an adaptive response from the CNS.

Several investigators report that visual and somatosensory deprivation delays or may ultimately limit vestibular compensation, although these effects appear to be species dependent and have yet to be satisfactorily determined in humans (Courjon, Jeannerod, Ossuzio, & Schmid, 1977; Lacour, Roll, & Appaix, 1976; Smith, Darlington, & Curthoys, 1986).

Some authors have described the short latency neuronal connections between the peripheral vestibular sensory receptors and the extraocular muscles that control eye movements as a simple three-neuron arc (Shepard & Telian, 1996). Discussions of this short latency network responsible for the VOR do not explain its adaptive capabilities when faced with an error signal.

Lisberger (1988) reports that the primitive nature of the three-neuron arc appears to allow for such short latencies in eye movement response to head movement. Any adaptation or recalibration in response to reduced visual acuity appears to take place higher in the brain stem. In other words, one part of the neural network is responsible for short latencies, and another part is responsible for accurate eye movements.

Gradual Reduction in Dynamic Asymmetry

As noted earlier, there is a gradual reduction in resting activity in the vestibular nuclei on both sides following unilateral vestibular deafferentation. With regard to dynamic symptoms, there is also a noted reduction in gain of the VOR in both directions immediately following unilateral labyrinthectomy (excision of the peripheral labyrinth). Over a period of days to weeks, there is a gradual increase in the gain of the VOR in response to head movements toward the *lesioned* side. The gain of the VOR for head movements toward the *intact* labyrinth remains reduced compared with its preoperative level. This increase of gain on the lesioned side and reduction in gain on the intact side result in a reduction in asymmetric response to horizontal head movements (Smith & Curthoys, 1989).

Restoration of VOR function plays a large role in the recovery of dynamic visual acuity following unilateral vestibular injury. For slow to moderate head movements, the intact labyrinth can provide sufficient stimulation to both vestibular nuclei to allow for adequate VOR response (and, therefore, clear vision). The inhibitory response from the intact labyrinth provides the necessary stimulus for these slow to moderate head movements. Due to the nonlinearity of

---

[2]Gain may be defined as the ratio of eye movement amplitude to head amplitude. A 10 degree head movement should result in a 10 degree eye movement in the opposite direction for a perfect gain of one.

the excitatory versus inhibitory responses of the sensory receptors (cristae) on the intact side, the faster the head movement, the less useful the inhibitory information from the intact side becomes when the head moves away from the intact side. There does not appear to be a measurable limit to the range of excitatory response, and the VOR responds normally to head movements toward the intact side up to 8 Hz. The inhibitory response saturates at zero spikes per second at moderate velocity head movements (around and above 200 degrees per second), which prohibits the intact labyrinth from accurately responding to faster head movements away from the intact side. Paige (1989) demonstrated that unilateral peripheral deficits could not be detected through rotational testing at these slower to moderate velocities. When the velocity of rotation was increased to 300 degrees per second, nonlinearities were consistently noted in patients that otherwise appeared fully compensated at four months post UVD. This deficit appears to be permanent and results in retinal slip with faster head movements toward the lesioned side (Curthoys & Halmagyi, 1996). This is the basis for head thrust testing (see Chapter 3).

Common Disorders of Vestibular and Balance Function

Benign Paroxysmal Positional Vertigo

By far, BPPV is the most common cause of episodic vertigo, and it has historically been found to be frequently misdiagnosed at the primary care level (Katsarkas, 1994; Li, Li, Epley, & Wienberg, 2000). Patients typically report brief episodes (less than 1 minute) of intense vertigo, usually brought on by lying down, rolling over in bed, or tilting the head back. BPPV is a mechanical dysfunction of the inner ear and does not usually represent an ongoing disease process. It is relatively easily diagnosed and treated. BPPV does not respond to medication; rather, it is most effectively treated by canalith repositioning procedures. The typical pattern of BPPV is one of intermittent episodes. The vertigo (spinning sensation) may occur frequently for weeks at a time, disappear for months, and then reappear with no warning.

BPPV is believed to be a result of a plug of calcium carbonate and protein crystals (otoconia) that have become dislodged from the utricle, settling most frequently in the posterior semicircular canal. Otoconia do not cause a problem until the patient moves in a manner that stimulates the offending semicircular canal. The otoconia then begin moving, causing abnormal stimulation of the motion sensor in the affected ear. While the otoconia are in motion (typically 15 to 45 seconds), the patient is experiencing conflicting signals from the two labyrinths of the inner ear.

By performing the Dix-Hallpike maneuver (see Chapter 3, Fig. 3–5) an episode of vertigo can often be elicited. If this maneuver makes the patient vertiginous, the eyes are simultaneously inspected for nystagmus. The direction of the nystagmus allows for identification of the specific offending canal. Once this has been accomplished, the patient can be treated. Websites offering additional information include www.familydoctor.org/handouts/200.html and www.bppvcure.com. A more detailed description of clinical signs associated with BPPV can be found in Chapter 3. Vestibular evaluation will usually result in a positive response (vertigo and nystagmus) to the Dix-Hallpike maneuver, although in some patients BPPV may not be active at the time of examination. If the history is suggestive of BPPV and the exam is negative, rescheduling the patient for repeat Dix-Hallpike testing is appropriate.

Vestibular Neuritis

Vestibular neuritis (also known as vestibular neuronitis) is characterized by a sudden onset of vertigo without any associated auditory symptoms. Vertigo is usually restricted to one attack, but a minority of patients may have repeated attacks (Bergenius & Perols, 1999). The vertigo is usually prolonged (lasting 24 hours or more) and is accompanied by nausea, vomiting, spontaneous nystagmus, and postural instability (Brandt, 1991). Vestibular neuritis is thought to be the result of a viral inflammation of the eighth nerve causing dysfunction of the superior division of the vestibular nerve. No specific virus has been deemed responsible; however, serology has demonstrated increased viral antibody titers to several viruses, including herpes simplex, Epstein-Barr, rubella, influenza, and cytomegalovirus (Bergenius & Perols, 1999). Acute symptoms can be reduced through the use of vestibular suppressant or antiemetic medications; however, gradual reduction of sedating medication and increased activity to promote central compensation are recommended (Brandt, 1991; Clendaniel & Helminski, 1993; Rubin, 1973; Zee, 1985).

Vestibular evaluation will usually demonstrate a caloric hypofunction on the affected side. Depending on the level of central compensation, direction-fixed nystagmus that reduces with visual fixation and reduced VOR gain on rotary tests may be noted.

Meniere's Disease

Meniere's disease is a disorder of the inner ear, which, in its classic presentation, is characterized by episodes of vertigo, unilateral decreased hearing, increased tinnitus, and aural fullness on the affected side. Its cause is unknown, but it is thought to be related to an inability of the ear to regulate endolymph, resulting in an episodic buildup of pressure in the membranous labyrinth.

The Committee on Hearing and Equilibrium of the American Academy of Otolaryngology defines Meniere's disease as an "idiopathic syndrome of endolymphatic hydrops." Endolymphatic hydrops varies greatly in both symptomology and duration and frequency of episodes. In the early stages of the disease, examination between episodes can be completely normal. As the disease progresses, decreased hearing and reduced vestibular sensitivity are typically noted in the affected ear. Variations of the disease have been described as "cochlear" or "vestibular" hydrops. In these conditions it is hypothesized that the isolated symptoms (fluctuating hearing OR episodic vertigo) are related to hydrops restricted to certain portions of the labyrinth (Andrews & Honrubia, 1996).

The diagnosis of Meniere's disease is based primarily on the patient's report of repeated episodes of the previously listed group of symptoms. Audiometric evaluation may reveal an asymmetrical, typically low-frequency sensorineural hearing loss. Vestibular evaluation typically demonstrates reduced vestibular function on the affected side. Inspection for nystagmus during an attack may reveal spontaneous nystagmus following Alexander's law (defined earlier in this chapter). Unlike other vestibular disorders, the nystagmus may beat (fast phase) toward the lesioned side. This is considered the result of increased vestibular output during the inflammatory process of a hydrops attack (Andrews & Honrubia, 1996). Vestibular evaluation will usually reveal a caloric hypofunction (defined in Chapter 5) on the affected side in patients with lengthy histories of episodic vertigo. In the early stages of the disease, caloric testing may be normal or even reveal a stronger caloric response in the pathologic ear due to inflammation of the labyrinth.

Perilymph Fistula

Perilymph fistulas (PF) are an abnormal communication between the perilymph (inner ear fluid) and the middle ear cavity. They are felt most often to be the result of barotrauma, head trauma, a complication of ear surgery, or excessive straining causing a sudden Valsalva maneuver (Brandt, 1991). To say that the diagnosis of PF is controversial is an understatement. There is no reliable test for PF, and even surgical exploration may result in vague findings. The standard treatment includes bed rest with the head elevated and avoidance of physical strain. Surgical treatment for patients with recurrent or prolonged symptoms consists of patching the most likely areas of fistulization (the round and oval windows) (Wall & Rauch, 1996).

Central Dizziness

Central dizziness is most often caused by a lesion in the cerebellum, brain stem, or central vestibular pathways. Sudden onset vertigo of central origin is more consistent with a vascular event such as infarction or ischemia. Progressive dizziness (imbalance or position-induced vertigo) accompanied by headache over a period of weeks to months is more suggestive of a space occupying tumor.

Vertebrobasilar insufficiency (VBI) is a specific type of central dizziness. The cause of VBI is thought to be atherosclerosis of the vertebral or basilar arteries. Symptoms include sudden onset vertigo lasting for several minutes, frequently accompanied by nausea and vomiting. Diagnosis is made by recognizing associated symptoms reflecting ischemia. The most common associated symptoms are incoordination, extremity weakness, confusion, headache, diplopia, and dysarthria (Baloh, 1996). Vestibular evaluation and neurologic evaluation are usually normal.

To be considered "central," the lesion must be located at or medial to the vestibular nuclei (Hirose & Halmagyi, 1996). If either of these is suspected, neurologic evaluation and neuroimaging are recommended. Vestibular evaluation may reveal abnormal oculomotor test scores, vertical nystagmus, or abnormally increased gain of the VOR on rotary tests.

Vestibular Equivalent Migraine

Vestibular migraine episodes follow the same temporal course as migraine headaches, which are quite varied. Patients typically complain of sudden onset rotary vertigo lasting anywhere from a few minutes to longer than 24 hours (Harker, 1996). They may or may not be associated with headache and typically are not accompanied by any associated auditory symptoms such as tinnitus, temporary hearing loss, or aural fullness. Some patients may complain of photophobia (hypersensitivity to light), phonophobia (hypersensitivity to sound), or scintillating scotoma (irregularly outlined luminous patch in the visual field). Vestibular migraines can be virtually indistinguishable from vestibular Meniere's disease (Tusa, 1999). Vestibular studies are usually normal, and diagnosis is achieved by clinical suspicion and positive response to prophylactic or abortive medical treatment used for migraine headaches.

Cervical Vertigo

Cervical vertigo (CV) is a controversial diagnosis, but it appears that some patients suffer vestibular type symptoms associated with neck tension or torsion. Symptoms of CV include lightheadedness, floating unsteadiness, and gait ataxia. (Brandt and Bronstein, 2001). Risk factors for CV include whiplash injury, cervical disc disease, degenerative arthritis, and repetitive motion stress injury. Vestibular evaluation will usually be normal; however, patients with CV may exhibit nystagmus with neck torsion. These patients generally do not respond to vestibular rehabilitation or medication. Referral to a physiatrist may be helpful.

Ototoxicity

Ototoxicity can occur after ingestion or exposure to substances toxic to the hair cells of the cochlea (cochleotoxic) or labyrinth (vestibulotoxic). The most frequent cause of ototoxicity is the administration of aminoglycoside antibiotics. Other medications such as loop diuretics, cisplatin, and high doses of aspirin can have ototoxic effects as well. It is particularly important for the primary care physician to be aware of potentiating effects of renal dysfunction and concomitant use of loop diuretics when considering the administration of aminoglycoside antibiotics.

Ototoxicity results in bilateral vestibular hypofunction. Patients typically do not complain of vertigo because the effects are bilateral, symmetrical, and gradual. Complaints associated with ototoxic bilateral vestibular hypofunction include gait instability and oscillopsia. Vestibular evaluation reveals bilateral hypofunction, often more severe in the lower frequencies, which can be demonstrated through caloric tests and rotary tests.

Acoustic Neuroma (Vestibular Schwannoma)

Acoustic neuromas are slow growing, benign encapsulated tumors that can arise in the cerebellopontine angle. The presenting symptom is usually unilateral hearing loss. Because of the slow growing nature of these tumors, loss of vestibular function is gradual and acute vertigo is not generally appreciated. Vestibular complaints are most often related to dysequilibrium. Diagnosis is best made through neuroimaging, specifically magnetic resonance imaging, with and without gadolinium enhancement (Hirose & Halmagyi, 1996). Vestibular evaluation usually demonstrates caloric hypofunction and sensorineural hearing loss on the affected side.

Mal de Debarquement Syndrome

In this poorly understood phenomenon, patients experience a persistent rocking sensation after spending time on a boat. Fortunately, these symptoms usually resolve within a few days. It is speculated that these patients have undergone some type of adaptation to the to-and-fro motion of the ship and have difficulty readapting to solid earth (Baloh, 1996). Occasionally, these symptoms can persist for month to years. Mal de Barquement syndrome is overwhelmingly more prevalent in females and in persistent cases does not appear to be responsive to vestibular suppressant medications. Benzodiazepines and vestibular therapy may provide some benefit (Murphy, 1993; Hain, Hanna, & Rheinberger, 1999).

Superior Canal Dehiscence Syndrome

This recently identified syndrome causes patients to experience vertigo and oscillopsia in response to loud noises or changes in middle ear pressure. High-resolution CT scanning has demonstrated "dehiscence of the bone overlying the superior semi-circular canal." Surgical plugging or resurfacing of the canal has relieved symptoms in the few patients that have undergone this procedure (Minor, 2000).

Barotrauma

Barotrauma can lead to relatively mild complaints of dysequilibrium thought to be associated with asymmetric middle ear pressure and can result in acute vertigo associated with perilymph fistula. These complaints are usually precipitated by an event involving extreme fluctuations in atmospheric pressure such as flying or scuba diving (Luxon, 1996).

Hyperventilation

See Chapter 3.

Postural (Orthostatic) Hypotension

See Chapter 3.

References

Allison, L. (1995). Balance disorders. In: D.A. Umphred (Ed.), *Neurologic rehabilitation* (pp. 802–837). St. Louis: Mosby-Yearbook.

Allum, H. J., & Pfaltz, C. R. (1985). Visual and vestibular contributions to pitch sway stabilization in the ankle muscles of normals and patients with bilateral peripheral vestibular deficits. *Exp Brain Res*, *58*, 82–94.

Andrews, J. C., & Honrubia, V. (1996). Meniere's disease. In: R. W. Baloh & G. M. Halmagyi (Eds.), *Disorders of the vestibular system* (pp. 300–317). New York: Oxford University Press.

Baloh, R. W. (1996). In: R. W. Baloh & G. M. Halmagyi (Eds.), *Disorders of the vestibular system* (pp. 157–170). New York: Oxford University Press.

Baloh, R. W., & Honrubia, V. (1990). *Clinical neurophysiology of the vestibular system*. Philadelphia: F.A. Davis.

Bergenius, J., & Perols, O. (1999). Vestibular neuritis: A follow up study. *Acta Otolaryngol*, *199*(8), 985–899.

Bienhold, H., & Flor, H. (1978). Role of commisural connections between vestibular nuclei in compensation following unilateral labyrinthectomy. *J Physiol*, *284*, 178P.

Bohmer, A. (1996). Acute unilateral peripheral vestibulopathy. In: R. W. Baloh & G. M. Halmagyi (Eds.), *Disorders of the vestibular system* (pp. 318–327). New York: Oxford University Press.

Brandt, T. (1991). Medical and physical therapy. In: T. Brandt (Ed.), *Vertigo: Its multisensory syndromes* (pp. 15–17). New York: Springer-Verlag.

Brandt, T., & Bronstein, A. M. (2001). Cervical vertigo. *J Neurol Neurosurg Psychiatry*, 71, 8–12.

Brown, J. J. (1993). A system oriented approach to the dizzy patient. In: I. K. Aranberg (Ed.), *Dizziness and balance disorders* (pp. 11–24). New York: Kugler Publications.

Carl, J. R. (1993). Practical anatomy and physiology of the ocular motor system. In: G. P. Jacobson, C. W. Newman, & J. M. Kartush (Eds.), *Handbook of balance function testing* (pp. 53–68). St. Louis: Mosby-Year Book.

Clendaniel, R. A., & Helminski, J. O. (1993). Rehabilitation strategies for patients with vestibular deficits. In: I. K. Arenberg (Ed.). *Dizziness and balance disorders* (pp. 663–667). New York: Kugler Publications.

Colledge, N. R., Cantley, P., Peaston, I., Brash, H., Lewis, S., & Wilson, J. A. (1994). Ageing and balance: The measurement of spontaneous sway by posturography. *Gerontology*, *40*, 273–278.

Courjon, J. H., Jeannerod, M., Ossuzio, I., & Schmid, R. (1977). The role of vision incompensation of vestibulo ocular reflex after hemilabyrinthectomy in the cat. *Exp Brain Res*, *28*, 235–248.

Curthoys, I. S., & Halmagyi, G. M. (1996). How does the brain compensate for vestibular lesions? In: R.W. Baloh & G. M. Halmagyi (Eds.), *Disorders of the vestibular system* (pp. 145–154). New York: Oxford University Press.

Demer, J. L., Honrubia, V., & Baloh, R. W. (1994). Dynamic visual acuity: a test for oscillopsia and vestibular-ocular reflex function. *Am J Otol*, *15*, 340–347.

Demer, J. L., Porter, F. I., Goldberg, J., Jenkins, H. A., Schmidt, K. (1989). Adaptation to telescopic spectacles: vestibulo-ocular reflex plasticity. *Invest Opthalmol Vis Sci*, *30*(1), 159–170.

Gonshor, A., & Melvill-Jones, G. (1976). Extreme vestibular ocular adaptation induced by prolonged optical reversal of vision. *J Physiol (Lond)*, *256*, 381–414.

Gresty, M. A., Hess, K., & Leech, J. (1977). Disorders of the vestibulo-ocular reflex producing oscillopsia and mechanisms compensating for loss of labyrinthine function. *Brain*, *100*, 693–716.

Gresty, M. A. (1996). Vestibular tests in evolution, I, Otolith testing. In: R. W. Baloh, & G. M. Halmagyi (Eds.), *Disorders of the vestibular system* (pp. 243–255). New York: Oxford University Press.

Hain, T. C., Hanna, P. A., & Rheinberger, M. A. (1999). Mal de Debarquement. *Arch Otolaryngol Head Neck Surg*, *125*(6), 615–620.

Hain, T. C., & Hillman, M. A. (1994). Anatomy and physiology of the normal vestibular system. In. S. J. Herdman (Ed.). *Vestibular rehabilitation* (pp. 3–20). Philadelphia: F.A. Davis.

Halmagyi, G. M., Colematch, J. G., & Curthoys, I. S. (1994). New tests of vestibular function. *Baillieres Clin Neurol*, *3*(3), 485–500.

Halmagyi, G. M., Gresty, M. A., & Gibson, W. P. R. (1979). Ocular tilt reaction with peripheral vestibular lesion. *Ann Neurol*, *6*, 80–83.

Harker, L. E. (1996). Migraine associated vertigo. In: R. W. Baloh & G. M. Halmagyi (Eds.), *Disorders of the vestibular system* (pp. 407–417). New York: Oxford University Press.

Highstein, S. M. (1996). How does the vestibular part of the inner ear work? In: R. W. Baloh, & S. M. Highstein (Eds.), *Disorders of the vestibular system* (pp. 3–11). New York: Oxford University Press.

Hirose, G., & Halmagyi, G. M. (1996). Brain tumors and balance disorders. In: R. W. Baloh & G. M. Halmagyi (Eds.), *Disorders of the vestibular system* (pp. 446–460). New York: Oxford University Press.

Hobeika, C. P. (1999). Equilibrium and balance in the elderly. *Ear Nose Throat J*, *78* (8), 558–566.

Honrubia, V., & Hoffman, L. F. (1993). Practical anatomy and physiology of the vestibular system. In: Jacobson, G. P., Newman, C. W., & Kartush, J. M. (Eds.), *Handbook of balance function testing* (pp. 9–52). St. Louis: Mosby Year Book.

Igarashi, M. (1984). Vestibular compensation: an overview. *Acta Otolaryngol (Stockh) Suppl*, *406*, 78–82.

JC. (1952). Living without a balancing mechanism. *N Engl J Med*, *246*, 458–460.

Katsarkas, A. (1994). Dizziness in aging: A retrospective study of 1194 cases. *Arch Otolaryngol Head Neck Surg*, *110* (3), 296–301.

Keshner, E. A. (1994). Postural abnormalities in vestibular disorders. In: S. J. Herdman (Ed.), *Vestibular rehabilitation* (pp. 47–67). Philadelphia: F.A. Davis.

Khater, T. T., Baker, J. F., & Peterson, B. W. (1990). Dynamics of adaptive change in human vestibulo-ocular reflex direction. *J Vestib Res*, *1*, 23–29.

Lacour, M., Roll, J. P., & Appaix, M. (1976). Modifications and development of spinal reflexes in the alert baboon (*Papio papio*) following an unilateral vestibular neurectomy. *Brain*, *113* (2), 255–269.

Leigh, R. J., & Zee, D. S. (1991). *The neurology of eye movements* (2nd ed.) Philadelphia: F.A. Davis.

Li, J. C., Li, C. J., Epley, J., & Wienberg, L. (2000). Cost effective management of benign positional vertigo using canalith repositioning. *Arch Otolaryngol Head Neck Surg*, *122* (3), 334–339.

Lisberger, S. (1988). The neural basis for learning of simple motor skills. *Science*, *242*, 728–735.

Longridge, N. S. & Mallinson, A. I. (1984). A discussion of the dynamic illegible "E" test: a new method of screening aminoglycoside vestibulotoxicity. *Arch Otolaryngol Head Neck Surg*, *92*, 671–677.

Luxon, L. (1996). Posttruamatic vertigo. In: R. W. Baloh, & G. M. Halmagyi (Eds.), *Disorders of the vestibular system* (pp. 381–395). New York: Oxford University Press.

Minor, L. B. (2000). Superior canal dehiscence syndrome. *Am J Otol*, *21* (1), 9–19.

Murphy, T. P. (1993). Mal de debarquement syndrome: a forgotten entity? *Otolaryngol Head Neck Surg*, *109* (1), 10–13.

Paige, G. D. (1989). Nonlinearity and asymmetry in the human vestibulo-ocular reflex. *Acta Otolaryngol*, *108*, 1–8.

Precht, W., Shimazu, H., & Markham, C. (1966). The problem of central compensation of vestibular function after hemilabyrinthectomy. *J Neurophysiol*, *29*, 996–1010.

Robinson, D., Zee, D. S., Hain, T. C., Holmes, A., & Rosenbug, L. (1984). Alexander's law: its behavior and origin in the human vestibule-ocular reflex. *Ann Neurol*, *16* (6), 714–722.

Rubin, W. (1973). Vestibular suppressant drugs. *Arch Otolaryngol*, 97, 135–138.

Sawyer, R. M., Thurston, S. E., Becker, K. R., Ackley, C. V., Seidman, S. H., & Leigh, J. R. (1994). The cervico-ocular reflex of normal human subjects in response to transient and sinusoidal trunk rotations. *J Vestib Res*, *4* (3), 245–249.

Shepard, N. T., & Telian, S. A. (1996). *Practical management of the balance disorder patient*. San Diego: Singular Publishing Group.

Smith, P. F., & Curthoys, I. S. (1989). Mechanisms of recovery following unilateral labyrinthectomy: a review. *Brain Res Rev*, *14*, 155–180.

Smith, P. F., Darlington, C. L., & Curthoys, I. S. (1986). The effect of visual deprivation on vestibular compensation in the guinea pig. *Brain Res*, *364*, 195–198.

Tusa, R. J. (1999, July). Migraine induced dizziness: diagnosis and management. *ENG Report*. Chicago: ICS Medical Corporation.

Wall, C., & Rauch, S. D. S. (1996). Perilymphatic fistula. In: R. W. Baloh & G. M. Halmagyi (Eds.), *Disorders of the vestibular system* (pp. 396–406). New York: Oxford University Press.

Wright, C. G., & Schwade, N. D. (2000). Anatomy and physiology of the vestibular system. In: R. J. Roeser, M. Valente, & H. Hossford-Dunn (Eds.), *Audiology diagnosis*. New York: Thieme Medical Publishers.

Zee, D. (1994). Vestibular adaptation. In: S. J. Herdman (Ed.), *Vestibular rehabilitation* (pp. 68–79). Philadelphia: F.A. Davis.

Zee, D. (1985). Perspectives on the pharmacotherapy of vertigo. *Arch Otolaryngol*, *111*, 609–612.

3

Screening Tests for Vestibular Dysfunction

The goal of the initial office examination is to determine whether the probable site of the lesion is peripheral or central. A directed case history and brief physical examination often allow a more direct route to diagnosis and treatment. The examiner is responsible for determining on initial contact whether the patient's complaints suggest a neurologic emergency such as brain stem stroke (Baloh, 1998). Once the examiner is comfortable that the patient's symptoms and physical signs are of a nonurgent nature, an examination to categorize the patient's "type" of dizziness follows.

Patients with chronic balance disorders typically see several different physicians without a diagnosis or resolution to their complaint. Many are treated symptomatically with vestibular suppressant medication even though a diagnosis of vestibular dysfunction has not been made. In many cases, patients with a chronic history of symptoms report that a thorough history was never taken (Linstrom, 1992). To quote Dr. Joel Goebel, "The accuracy and quality of the history is directly related to the patience and skill of the examiner" (personal communication). It is therefore important to spend sufficient time with individual patients to understand their history and complaints thoroughly before attempting to make a diagnosis.

Role of the Case History Interview

A thorough history is critical for three main reasons:

1. Many patients have difficulty articulating their symptoms beyond simply describing themselves as being "dizzy."
2. Additional evaluation and treatment will differ depending on the suspected site of the lesion.
3. Some vestibular disorders cannot be differentiated solely on the results of vestibular evaluation (e.g., Meniere's disease versus labyrinthitis) (Shepard, 1999).

45

The value of a thorough history should not be underestimated. This is reflected in the result of one study in which a provisional diagnosis based only on case history and screening examinations proved correct for 76% of patients seen (Kroenke et al., 1992).

Preexamination Preparations

Before the initial patient appointment, it is important that the patient be sent a questionnaire with instructions to complete it before arriving for the appointment. The questionnaire is not intended to be a substitute for a comprehensive case history interview but rather as a motivation for the patient to think about how to articulate the symptoms. The questionnaire should focus not only on current symptoms but also on the patient's recalling the first episode of dizziness. It should also include questions about associated symptoms that the patient may not consider part of the "dizziness problem" (Fig. 3–1).

Structure of the Case History Interview

The case history interview should be initially unstructured and open ended. Patients should be allowed to tell their story with minimal interruption. One approach is to ask the patient, "Tell me, what brings you here?" It is helpful to ask patients to start at the beginning and present their story chronologically. Patients should be asked to present their symptoms as they experience them and to avoid using any medical diagnoses they may have been given. Once patients have presented their own interpretation of the symptoms, a review of previous medical testing and treatment can help to prevent duplication of testing.

After giving patients an opportunity to describe the symptoms in their own words, a series of pointed questions to gain additional details is usually required. Although most patients respond appropriately to the questions, some need to be refocused frequently and instructed to listen closely to the question being asked, restricting the answers to addressing only their specific question. Using the questionnaire as a guide, it is the job of the examiner to extract the necessary information from the patient in an effort to categorize the patient's "type" of dizziness before beginning any examination. Information should be obtained regarding the quality and temporal course of symptoms; precipitating, exacerbating, and relieving factors; associated symptoms; and the patient's general health status.

Quality

The key to a preliminary diagnosis is determining whether the patient's complaints are of vertigo. Vertigo is described as a sensation or illusion of spinning or rotation, continuing with the eyes closed. Vertigo indicates the strong likelihood of peripheral vestibular disease, but central disease cannot be ruled out. Motion-provoked dysequilibrium and nausea are frequently associated with a nonacute vestibular loss. Other frequent descriptions of symptoms include

Figure 3–1. Dizziness History Questionnaire Sample

Name:_____ Age:_____ Date:_____

WHEN was the first time ever in your life you had dizziness?

_____

WHAT were the circumstances?

_____

_____

WHEN was the last time you experienced dizziness?

_____

WHAT were the circumstances?

_____

_____

Currently, my dizziness...(Check <u>ONE</u>)
__ is constant.
__ is always there, but changes in intensity.
__ comes and goes.
If it comes and goes:
How long does it typically last? ___ seconds / minutes / hours (Circle <u>ONE</u>)
How often does it typically occur? ___ times per hour/day/week/month/year
My dizziness mostly consists of... (Check <u>ALL</u> that apply)
__ spells of spinning with nausea.
__ off-balance sensation without dizziness.
__ a light-headed or near faint sensation.
__ other. Please explain

_____

Between episodes I feel... (Check <u>ONE</u>)
__ dizzy or off balance all the time.
__ normal.
__ other. Please explain

_____

My episodes occur... (Check <u>ALL</u> that apply)
__ spontaneously. Nothing I do seems to bring them on or turn them off.
__ only when standing or walking.
__ in relation to any head motion.
__ in relation to only certain head positions. Please describe

_____

When I roll over in bed... (Check <u>ONE</u>)
__ nothing unusual happens.
__ the room seems to spin sometimes.
__ the room spins every time.

Is there anything that you can do to make your dizziness go away? (sit, lay down, close eyes. . .)
Please explain:

___

Circle all that apply:
I have hearing difficulty ....Right .....Left .....Both
I have ringing or other sounds ....Right .....Left .....Both
I have fullness ....Right .....Left .....Both
I have had ear surgery ....Right .....Left .....Both
Circle YES or NO
Did you have a cold, flu, or virus type symptoms shortly before the onset of your dizziness?   YES / NO
Did you cough, lift, sneeze, fly in a plane, swim under water, have a head trauma shortly before the onset of your dizziness?   YES / NO
If you had head trauma prior to your dizziness, did you lose consciousness completely?   YES / NO
Were you exposed to any irritating fumes, paints, etc. at the onset of your dizziness?   YES / NO
Do you get dizzy when you have not eaten for a long time?   YES / NO
Did you get new glasses recently?   YES / NO
I consider myself to be an anxious or tense type of person. . .   YES / NO
I am under a great deal of stress. . .   YES / NO
In the past year I have had. . . (Check <u>ALL</u> that apply)
__ loss of consciousness   __ occasional loss of vision
__ seizures or convulsions   __ severe pounding headache or migraine
__ slurring of speech   __ palpitations of the heartbeat
__ difficulty swallowing   __ tingling around mouth
__ weakness in one hand, arm or leg   __ tendency to fall
__ double vision   __ loss of balance when walking
__ spots before the eyes
I have or have had. . . (Check <u>ALL</u> that apply)
__ Diabetes   __ Stroke
__ High blood pressure   __ Migraine headaches
__ Arthritis   __ A neck and/or back injury
__ Irregular heartbeat   __ Allergies
**Please check below for any MEDICATIONS you have tried
or are currently taking for dizziness:**

	Taken in past	Taking now	Helps
Antivert (meclizine)	___	___	___
Valium (diazepam)	___	___	___
Dyazide "water pills"	___	___	___

Have you ever been previously evaluated for dizziness?

___

___

lightheadedness, dysequilibrium while stationary, or "feeling drunk." These complaints are often associated with systemic or central nervous system (CNS) disease.

Some patients with vestibular dysfunction describe their symptoms in a vague manner. Patients with partially compensated vestibular dysfunction may describe situational anxiety and disorientation. For example, many patients with vestibular weakness will describe a sensation of disorientation and anxiety while walking in a crowded area such as a shopping mall, particularly when walking against traffic. In this situation, the patient's visual field is moving, making it unreliable for judging relative motion. A sense of disorientation or fear may overcome the uncompensated patient. This can easily be misinterpreted as, or may eventually become, an anxiety-producing event leading to agoraphobia.

Patients with vestibular dysfunction develop an increased reliance on visual information for the maintenance of balance. They are subject to an optokinetic effect when walking down the aisle of a store (Ell, 1992), during which the eye is involuntarily drawn to objects in the periphery of the visual field. This phenomenon has been described as "supermarket syndrome." Optokinetic tracking is, for the most part, involuntary. Different colored objects on the shelves can create an optokinetic effect similar to that perceived during sustained horizontal rotation, and a sense of dysequilibrium or spatial disorientation will ensue. The common denominator of these situations is the "decreased visual input for orientation in space" (Jacob, 1988).

Temporal Course

Temporal course includes information regarding the onset, duration, and frequency of symptoms. In general, dizziness lasting for less than 1 minute when the patient is lying down is associated with benign paroxysmal positional vertigo (BPPV), whereas dizziness lasting less than 1 minute when the patient is standing is associated with orthostatic hypotension.

Dizziness lasting several minutes is most often associated with peripheral vestibular disorders, but it can be associated with vascular etiology, such as migraines or transient ischemic attacks. Dizziness lasting hours with a gradual decrease of symptoms is associated with unilateral peripheral vestibular disease, such as labyrinthitis, neuronitis, or hydrops (Meniere's syndrome). Dizziness of more than 24-hours' duration without a gradual decrease of symptoms may be associated with CNS or psychiatric disease.

Distinct episodes or sudden onset of symptoms suggests peripheral disease, whereas gradual onset is indicative of a more central disorder. Patients with BPPV often report constant dizziness over a period of hours to days. It is important to address these statements with further inquiry as to whether the vertigo was constant or experienced only when the patient moved his or her head during the specified time.

Many patients describe the duration of their symptoms as "quite a while" or "not too long." These patients should be instructed to be specific by using seconds and minutes to describe the duration of symptoms.

Precipitating, Exacerbating, or Relieving Factors

Symptoms that are brought on or increased by a change in head position, or with eyes closed, suggest peripheral disease. Symptoms noticed only while standing, but never when sitting or lying, suggest vascular or orthopedic disease. Symptoms that are constant and are unaffected by position change are suggestive of central pathology.

Associated Symptoms

Symptoms such as tinnitus, hearing loss, otalgia, or aural fullness, particularly unilateral complaints, suggest the probability of peripheral vestibular disease. Symptoms such as slurred speech, syncope or presyncope, numbness or tingling of the face or extremities, or "spots before eyes" suggest a more central etiology.

General Health Status

Patients with advanced diabetes may exhibit dysequilibrium and postural instability secondary to peripheral neuropathy or may experience postural hypotension secondary to autonomic neuropathy. Patients with a history of cardiovascular disease may experience reduced blood volume to the brain. Patients with a history of migraine headache are prone to vestibular migraine.

Medications

A review of the patient's current and past medications is useful in the case history interview. Not only does this provide the examiner insight as to possible medication-related dizziness or vertigo, it also provides a second chance to review any health conditions that the patient may have omitted from the history interview.

Smith (1991) reports that *The Physicians' Desk Reference* lists nearly a thousand medications with dizziness or a related complaint listed as a possible side effect. Skiendzielewski and Martyak (1980) reported that between 10 and 20% of patients presenting to an emergency room for dizziness were experiencing these symptoms as a result of medications. Past use of ototoxic medication, such as aminoglycoside antibiotics, and certain chemotherapy agents should be explored. Because most patients are unfamiliar with the exact medications used, it is typically more productive to inquire about treatment for certain conditions. For example, an inquiry about the use of aminoglycoside antibiotics could be phrased, "Have you ever been treated with intravenous antibiotics?" Inquiry into the use of chemotherapy agents could be phrased, "Have you ever been treated for cancer?" Because these medications are typically reserved for life-threatening conditions, it is not unusual for the patient to be completely unaware of their potential ototoxic effects. Whether the patient was not informed by the physician or was simply too focused on overall health to be concerned about side effects is a subject of speculation.

Table 3–1. Drug-Associated Eye-Movement Disorders

Drugs	Eye movement Disorders
Alcohol (ethanol)	Vestibular dysfunction: positional nystagmus Brain stem–cerebellar dysfunction pattern
Aminoglycoside antibiotics Streptomycin Gentamicin	Vestibular dysfunction: permanent Labyrinthine Hypofunction
Anticonvulsants Dilantin (phenytoin) Tegretol (carbamazepine)	Brain stem–cerebellar dysfunction pattern
Antidepressants Tricyclics (e.g., Elavil) Phenothiazines (e.g., Pamelor) Others (e.g., Prozac) Lithium	Central sedation pattern Internuclear ophthalmoplegia Opsoclonus Partial or total gaze paresis Brain stem–cerebellar pattern Opsoclonus
Chemotherapeutic anticancer agents (e.g., cisplatin)	Vestibular dysfunction: permanent Labyrinthine hypofunction
Diuretics Lasix Ethacrynic acid	Vestibular dysfunction: transient Labyrinthine hypofunction
Haldol (haloperidol)	Opsoclonus
Industrial solvents XyleneTrichloroethylene	Brain stem–cerebellar dysfunction pattern Vestibular dysfunction: central positional nystagmus Exaggerated VOR
Marijuana	Brain stem–cerebellar dysfunction pattern
Methadone	Brain stem–cerebellar dysfunction pattern
Quinine	Vestibular dysfunction: positional nystagmus
Salicylates Aspirin (acetylsalicylic acid)	Vestibular dysfunction: transient Labyrinthine hypofunction
Stimulants Amphetamine	Impaired accommodation/convergence: Reduced saccadic latency
Sedatives Barbiturates (e.g., phenobarbital, seconal) Chloral hydrate	Brain stem–cerebellar dysfunction pattern Vestibular dysfunction: central positional nystagmus

Tobacco	Upbeat nystagmus
Smoking or chewing nicotine gum	Square-wave jerks
Tranquilizers	Central sedation pattern
Benzodiazepines (e.g., Valium,	Brain stem – cerebellar pattern
Ativan, Xanax)	
Vestibular suppressants	Central sedation pattern
Meclizine	Vestibular dysfunction: transient
Benadryl	Labyrinthine hypofunction
Scopolamine	
Phenergan	
Flunarizine	

Reprinted with permission from Cass, S., & Furman, J. (1993, Nov). Medications and their effects on vestibular function testing. In: *ENG report* (pp. 81–84). Chicago: ICS Medical

Medications and Vestibular Testing

Many medications can affect the sensitivity and accuracy of vestibular testing. Antidepressants, sedatives and tranquilizers, and vestibular suppressants can cause test results suggestive of cerebellar or brain stem pathology. Diuretics, particularly Lasix (furosemide), can cause transient vestibular hypofunction. Alcohol, marijuana, and aspirin ingested within 24 hours of the examination can lead to spurious results (Cass & Furman, 1993). In addition to the effects noted in Table 3–1, alcohol, in sufficient quantities, can cause gaze-evoked nystagmus. It is best to have the patient avoid any of these medications for 48 hours before vestibular evaluation. If this is not possible, interpretation regarding CNS signs must be made with caution. Cass and Furman (1993) offer a thorough review of potential artifacts that can result from the use of certain medications while undergoing vestibular evaluation (Table 3–1).

Examination of the Vestibular Ocular Reflex

For most peripheral labyrinthine or "central" neurologic diseases, the eyes are the windows to the vestibular system. Inspection of eye movements can provide considerable information to assist in preliminary diagnosis. The two categories of eye movement are (1) reflexive eye movements generated by stimulation of the peripheral vestibular apparatus and (2) voluntary eye movements controlled by the cerebellum. Certain patterns of nystagmus are associated with either peripheral labyrinthine or central site of lesion.

Static Evaluation

Static evaluation of vestibular dysfunction primarily involves inspection for spontaneous or gaze nystagmus. These are best viewed through Frenzel lenses or infrared video oculography (see Chapter 4 for photographs and more information about these observation techniques), but can be viewed directly with the help of a penlight, otoscope, or ophthalmoscope.

Spontaneous or gaze nystagmus represents a tonic imbalance in the vestibular system. Peripheral vestibular nystagmus is horizontal rotary, whereas pure vertical or pure torsional nystagmus is considered a sign of central etiology. Peripheral vestibular nystagmus diminishes with visual fixation, whereas central nystagmus is not affected by fixation and may even increase. Peripheral vestibular nystagmus is mostly conjugate, whereas central nystagmus may be more intense in one eye. Peripheral vestibular nystagmus will increase in intensity when gaze is directed toward the fast phase (typically away from the lesion side) and will decrease with gaze away from the fast phase. Central nystagmus may have a change in the direction of the fast phase when gaze is shifted (Busis, 1993).

Dynamic Evaluation

HEADSHAKE NYSTAGMUS

Headshake nystagmus (HSN) is believed to be a result of dynamic asymmetry within the vestibular ocular reflex (VOR). As the head is shaken back and forth in a horizontal fashion, the intact labyrinth is generating a stronger response than the lesioned side. This increase in activity on the intact side builds up and is stored in a "central velocity storage mechanism." When the headshaking ceases, this stored energy discharges, causing a slow-phase response away from the intact labyrinth, resulting in a brief period of nystagmus beating away from the lesioned labyrinth.

Evaluation for HSN can be done through direct visualization, electro-oculography, or infrared video monitoring. Goebel and Garcia (1992) report that HSN can be easily documented using Frenzel lenses. The patient is instructed to tilt his or her head down at 30 degrees and then to shake the head back and forth as quickly as possible for a period of 30 seconds. This can also be done manually by the examiner.

Immediately following cessation of movement, the eyes are opened and observed for nystagmus. A brief period of horizontal nystagmus may be noted. Three patterns of post-HSN have been identified. The most common is a brief horizontal nystagmus beating away from the lesioned labyrinth, which occurs within the first several seconds following headshake. A second pattern involves a horizontal nystagmus beating toward the lesioned side and occurring about 20 seconds after the headshake. This is felt to be a central compensatory response and is termed recovery *nystagmus*. A third pattern involves both the aforementioned types with an initial burst of nystagmus away from the lesioned side, then a reversal in direction toward the lesioned side. Again, this is believed to be the result of a compensatory response to peripheral vestibular asymmetry (Jacobson, Newman, & Safadi, 1990).

The presence of HSN correlates well with peripheral vestibular function; however, HSN has been identified in patients with cerebellar dysfunction. HSN secondary to central lesions may exhibit a vertical component following a horizontal headshake maneuver (Zee & Fletcher, 1996). Jacobson et al. (1990)

report that HSN testing has a low sensitivity (27%) but fairly good specificity (85%) for identifying patients with vestibular dysfunction. They note that a potential weakness of their study is the fact that their "gold standard" for identifying patients with vestibular dysfunction was through caloric and rotary chair testing. Neither of these tests evaluates the high-frequency area (≥ 1 to 2 Hz) of the VOR thought to be involved in the generation of headshake nystagmus.

HEAD THRUST (HEAD IMPULSE) TEST

The VOR in response to head movement may be evaluated by rotating the patient's head in the YAW plane (as in shaking the head "no"), first at slower speeds to allow the patient time to become familiar with the procedure and relax

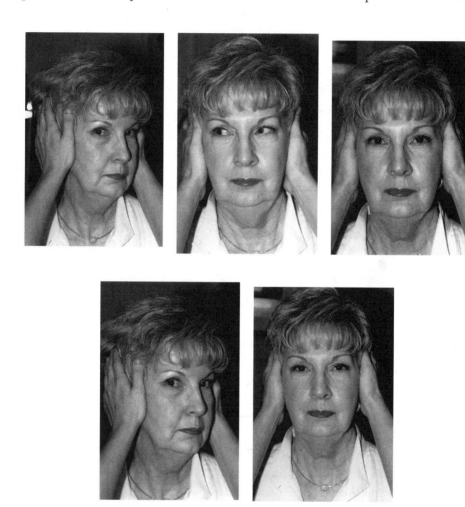

Figure 3–2. (Top row) A patient loses fixation on the focal point when her head is moved toward the affected side, requiring a catch-up corrective saccade to regain fixation. (Bottom row) A patient maintains fixation on the focal point. This is considered a "normal

the muscles in the neck. Start with the patient's head 15 to 30 degrees lateral from center. The patient's eyes should be focused on a centered target, typically on the examiner's nose. Then apply brief, high-acceleration head thrusts of about 15 to 30 degrees back to center (Fig. 3–2). The examiner should monitor the patient's eye movements to see whether visual fixation is maintained or whether the patient loses visual contact and must make quick corrective eye movements (catch-up saccades) to gain visual contact with the target (Harvey, Wood, & Feroah, 1997).

Horizontal head movement tests the horizontal semicircular canal, whereas the anterior and posterior canals can be tested by rotating the head in a diagonal direction (Cremer et al., 1998). A lack of visual fixation and subsequent catch-up saccade during rapid head acceleration suggest a loss of function in the corresponding ipsilateral semicircular canal (Aw et al., 1999). For example, a loss of visual fixation with a rapid horizontal head thrust to the right would be consistent with decreased sensitivity in the right horizontal semicircular canal, as shown in Fig. 3–2.

DYNAMIC VISUAL ACUITY

Another simple test of the VOR is to have the patient read a Snellen eye chart (Fig. 3–3) and establish visual acuity. This is followed by the examiner rotating the patient's head back and forth at a speed of 1 and 2 Hz horizontally while

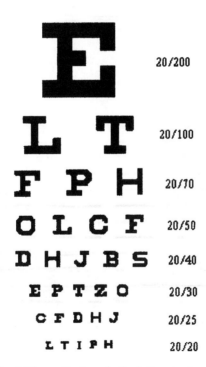

E	20/200
L T	20/100
F P H	20/70
O L C F	20/50
D H J B S	20/40
E P T Z O	20/30
C F D H J	20/25
L T I P H	20/20

Figure 3–3. Snellen eye chart: The patient reads the letters in descending order to establish static visual acuity.

reading the chart. Loss of one line is considered normal. Loss of three lines indicates possible VOR deficit (Longridge & Mallinson, 1987). Scoring visual acuity is usually determined by noting the lowest line on which the patient cannot correctly identify at least 50% of the optotypes (characters).

Sensitivity and specificity in testing dynamic visual acuity may be improved using recently developed computerized measurement techniques. Using these techniques, static visual acuity is measured, and the patient is then instructed to rotate his or her head in a sinusoidal back and forth motion in the YAW plane. Speed or velocity of head motion is measured using the same type of motion sensor used in active head rotation testing (see Fig. 3–4). The characters on the screen are visible only when the patient's head is moving above a preset speed. To evaluate effectively the contribution of the VOR to dynamic visual acuity, the speed of head movement must exceed the limits of the voluntary pursuit system, typically the upper limit of which approaches 2 Hz. To provide additional information to help lateralize vestibular dysfunction, the software can be adjusted to allow the characters to be visible only when the head is moving in a single direction. Herdman et al. (1998) reports that this technique is highly sensitive and specific for differentiating normal patients from patients with vestibular dysfunction.

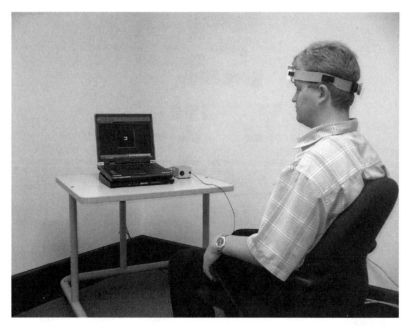

Figure 3–4. Dynamic visual acuity: The patient moves his head back and forth while viewing the computer screen. When the speed of head movement exceeds a predetermined level, a character appears on the screen. If the head slows down to below the predetermined speed, the character disappears.

Eye-Movement Tests

These tests of voluntary control of eye movements provide information about the patient's ability to perform efficient and accurate eye movements that are controlled by the cerebellum (Leigh & Zee, 1991). Although the age of the patient must be taken into consideration when assessing what is "normal," gross abnormalities on eye-movement tests indicate the possibility of CNS disease and referral for neurologic evaluation.

Saccadic tracking can be assessed by having the patient quickly shift the gaze from one point to another, typically the examiner's nose and a finger held out to the side. Accuracy, speed, and initiation time should be judged. Smooth pursuit can be tested by having the patient follow the examiner's finger as it moves slowly through the field of vision. Age, medications, and inattention can influence smooth pursuit ability; however, asymmetric or grossly abnormal responses indicate the possibility of cerebellar dysfunction.

Positioning

The *Dix-Hallpike maneuver* is performed to elicit nystagmus and vertigo commonly associated with BPPV. The patient is seated on an examining table and then, with the head turned 45 degrees to the side, is brought backwards rapidly into the supine position (Fig. 3–5). Most BPPV involves the posterior semicircular canal, and a positive response to this maneuver is the elicitation of vertigo and nystagmus that is rotary and beats upward and toward the undermost ear. There is usually a short latency (2 to 15 seconds) before the vertigo and nystagmus occur, and the duration of the signs is usually 15 to 45 seconds.

On having the patient rise quickly to the sitting position, a milder vertigo may be appreciated with nystagmus typically opposite that noted in the supine

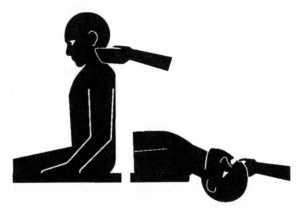

Figure 3–5. Dix-Hallpike maneuver: With the head turned and extended over the end of the examining table, the head should be turned both to the right and the left. (Reprinted with permission from Desmond, A. L., & Touchette, D. (1998). *Balance disorders: Evaluation and treatment: a short course for primary care physicians*. Chatham, IL: Micromedical Technologies.)

position. Repeated maneuvers result in reduced vertigo and nystagmus response. The examiner must be careful to note whether the nystagmus is purely vertical or persistent because these are indications of possible central nystagmus. BPPV can occur in the horizontal or anterior semicircular canals, and the duration and direction of the nystagmus will vary accordingly (Lempert & Tiel-Wick, 1996). (See Chapter 5 for details.)

Other Screening Examinations

Romberg Testing

The Romberg is a screening test for standing balance and is performed by having the patient stand with the feet together, arms either folded across the chest or at the sides. If the patient is able to maintain this position with minimal swaying, the patient is then asked to continue standing with eyes closed. Excessive sway with eyes closed relative to open may indicate a vestibular lesion, most often on the side to which the patient sways the most. Equal but excessive sway in the eyes open and eyes closed condition indicates possible proprioceptive weakness.

A tandem or sharpened Romberg can be performed by having the patient stand heel to toe and evaluating the postural stability with eyes open versus closed. This is simply a more difficult version of the Romberg test, and the interpretation would be similar. Patients with compensated vestibular dysfunction will often perform normally on the Romberg test, whereas patients with proprioceptive loss will exhibit the greatest difficulty. It is imperative to provide assurance that the examiner will not let the patient fall.

Dysdiadochokinesis Testing

Dysdiadochokinesis is the inability to make finely coordinated antagonistic movements. It is frequently seen in patients with cerebellar dysfunction. Testing for dysdiadochokinesis can be performed by having the patient perform rapid supination and pronation of the hands against the knees (rapid alternating hand movements). Poor performance on this test is believed to be the result of inappropriate timing of muscle activity disabling the patient from quickly stopping movement. This becomes visibly apparent when attempting to perform rapid alternating movements requiring efficient initiation and cessation of movement (Urbscheit & Oremland, 1995).

Tandem Gait Test

Tandem gait (walking heel to toe) in a tight figure eight or circular pattern requires an intact cerebellar function. An ataxic gait has been reported as the most common symptom of cerebellar dysfunction and is felt to be a result of the patient's inability to estimate the amount of muscle movement required to make a step (Urbscheit & Ormland, 1995). Because there are many causes other than cerebellar dysfunction for poor performance on tandem walking tasks, the specificity of this examination is understandably low.

Fukuda Stepping Test

This test involves having the patient march in place, with the eyes closed, for 100 steps. According to Fukuda (1959), normal patients are able to complete the task without moving more than 1 m or rotating more than 45 degrees. Patients with vestibular dysfunction reportedly deviate from center and frequently rotate in the direction of the affected labyrinth. Fukuda recommends that a grid be drawn on the floor, but simple observation can provide information about the patient's ability to remain oriented when visual and somatosensory feedback is diminished (Allison, 1995).

Screening for Hyperventilation Syndrome

Hyperventilation is more of an anxiety disorder than a vestibular disorder; however, many of these patients' primary complaints are of dizziness or lightheadedness, which they feel is unprovoked. Many of these patients are unaware of any coexisting symptoms until questioned by a clinician. Hyperventilation occurs when "ventilatory effort exceeds metabolic need" and causes hypocapnia (low level of arterial pCO_2), leading to constriction of the cerebral blood vessels and reduction of cerebral blood flow. Typical signs and symptoms include complaints of lightheadedness, frequent sighing, chest pain, and numbness and tingling around the mouth and hands. Some of these symptoms can be reproduced during examination in affected patients.

Anxiety can lead to increased heart rate and respirations, which can lead to hyperventilation. Drachman and Hart (1972) report that hyperventilation contributed to complaints of dizziness in 25 of 104 patients evaluated and was the sole cause in four patients. Sama, Meikle, & Jones (1995) report similar results stating that hyperventilation caused dizziness in 5% of subjects and was a contributing factor in another 21%. Sama et al. (1995) estimate that 65% of cases of hyperventilation are psychogenic, 31% mixed organic and psychogenic, and only 3% are pure organic.

Historically, the diagnosis of hyperventilation syndrome has been made by having the patient voluntarily overbreathe for a period of 90 seconds to 3 minutes. If the patient's symptoms were reproduced, a diagnosis of hyperventilation syndrome (HVS) was made (Vansteenkiste, Rochette, & Demedts, 1991). Recent studies indicate, however, that this hyperventilation provocation test has both poor sensitivity and poor specificity. Hornsveld, Garssen, Dop, & Van Speigel (1990) report that there was no difference in symptom reproduction in a group of suspected HVS patients compared with the results of voluntary overbreathing and response to mental overloading using a stressful mental tasking procedure. Similarly, Hornsveld and Garssen (1996) report that reproduction of symptoms did not differ in two groups of patients suspected of suffering from HVS: Group 1 was asked to overbreathe for a period of 3 minutes; group 2 followed the same instructions; however, CO_2 was titrated through a breathing mask to prevent hypocapnia.

Hanashiro (1990) warns that symptoms of hyperventilation can be produced by certain cardiovascular conditions and that patients presenting with these symptoms should undergo full medical evaluation before determining that these symptoms are the result of a benign anxiety disorder. The potential danger of having these patients voluntarily hyperventilate is that they may be experiencing symptoms secondary to decreased oxygen. Asking these patients to hyperventilate can further reduce the amount of oxygen in the bloodstream. Hyperventilation syndrome screening should not be performed in patients with significant cardiovascular or breathing problems. In most cases, symptom reproduction through hyperventilation infers that the patient's symptoms probably are not related to peripheral labyrinthine dysfunction. This does not mean, however, that vestibular studies should not be completed. Leigh and Zee (1991) report that occasionally hyperventilation will result in nystagmus associated with multiple sclerosis, acoustic neuroma, or vestibular neuritis. They hypothesize that hyperventilation may improve nerve conduction and temporarily increase the tonic discharge from the affected auditory nerve, resulting in asymmetric discharge and nystagmus.

Testing for Orthostatic (Postural) Hypotension

Many patients complain of dizziness or lightheadedness on rising from the sitting or supine position. Postural dizziness has been loosely correlated with postural or orthostatic hypotension. The American Academy of Neurology (1996) has issued a consensus statement defining orthostatic hypotension:

> Orthostatic hypotension (OH) is a reduction of systolic blood pressure of at least 20 mm Hg or diastolic blood pressure of at least 10 mm Hg within three minutes of standing. It is a physical sign and not a disease. An acceptable alternative to standing is the demonstration of a similar drop in blood pressure within three minutes, using a tilt table in the head up position, at an angle of at least 60 degrees. Confounding variables to be considered when reaching a diagnosis should include: food ingestion, time of day, state of hydration, ambient temperature, recent recumbency, postural deconditioning, hypertension, medications, gender, and age. Orthostatic hypotension may be symptomatic or asymptomatic. Symptoms of OH are those that develop on assuming the erect posture or following head-up tilt and usually resolve on resuming the recumbent position. They may include lightheadedness, dizziness, blurred vision, weakness, fatigue, cognitive impairment, nausea, palpitations, tremulousness, headache and neck ache. If the patient has symptoms suggestive of, but does not have documented, orthostatic hypotension, repeated measurements of blood pressure should be performed. Occasional patients may not manifest significant falls in blood pressure until they stand for at least ten minutes." (American Academy of Neurology, 1996)

Orthostatic hypotension is not uncommon in patients taking medication for hypertension or cardiac disease or in patients with autonomic nervous system neuropathy secondary to diabetes. Postural dizziness (dizziness on rising) and postural hypotension are common in the older population but are not highly correlated with each other. The cause of postural dizziness without concomitant postural hypotension is unknown, but some researchers have suggested a temporary impairment of cerebral blood flow (Stark & Wodak, 1983; Wollner, McCarthy, Soper, & Macy, 1979), as part of an "autonomic dysregulation" syndrome (Nozawa, Imamura, Hisamatsu, & Murakami, 1996.)

Orthostatic hypotension can be evaluated by having the patient lie down for 5 to 10 minutes and then checking blood pressure while still in the supine position. The examiner then asks the patient to stand up quickly, and then the examiner rechecks the blood pressure immediately and again after about 1 minute (Puiseux et al., 1999).

References

Allison, L. (1995). Balance disorders. In: D. Umphred (Ed.), *Neurologic rehabilitation*, 3rd ed. (pp. 802– 837). St. Louis: Mosby-Year Book.

American Academy of Neurology. American Autonomic Society, Consensus Committee. (1996). Consensus statement on the definition of orthostatic hypotension, pure autonomic failure, and multiple system atrophy. *Neurology*, 46, 1470.

Aw, S. T., Halmagyi, G. M., Black, R. A., Curthoys, I. S., Yavor, R. A., & Todd, M. J. (1999). Head impulses reveal loss of individual semicircular canal function. *J Vestib Res*, 9, 173– 180.

Baloh, R. (1998). Dizziness: Neurological emergencies. *Neurol Clin North Am*, 16(2), 305– 321.

Busis, S. N. (1993). Office evaluation of the dizzy patient. In: I. K. Arenberg (Ed.), *Dizziness and balance disorders* (pp. 159– 173). New York: Kugler Publications.

Cass, S., & Furman, J. (1993, Nov). Medications and their effects on vestibular function testing. In: *ENG report* (pp. 81– 84). Chicago: ICS Medical.

Cremer, P., Halmagyi, G. M., Aw, S. T., Curthoys, I. S., McGarvie, L.A., Todd, M.J., et al. (1998). Semicircular canal plane head impulses detect absent function of individual semicircular canals. *Brain*, 121, 699– 716.

Desmond, A. L. (2000). Vestibular rehabilitation. In: M. Valente, H. Hosford-Dunn, & R. J. Roeser (Eds.), *Audiology treatment* (pp. 639– 676). New York: Thieme Medical Publishers.

Desmond, A. L., & Touchette, D. (1998). *Balance disorders: Evaluation and treatment: A short course for primary care physicians*. Chatham, IL: Micromedical Technologies.

Drachman, D. A., & Hart, C. W. (1972). An approach to the dizzy patient. *Neurology*, 22, 323– 333.

Ell, J. (1992). Dizziness— organic or functional? *Aust Fam Physician*, 21(10), 1431– 1436.

Faye, E. E. (1976). *Clinical low vision*. Boston: Little, Brown and Company.

Fukuda, T. (1959). The stepping test: Two phases of the labyrinthine reflex. *Acta Otolaryngol*, 50, 95.

Goebel, J., & Garcia, P. (1992). Prevalence of post-headshake nystagmus in patients with caloric deficits and vertigo. *Otolaryngol Head Neck Surg*, 106(2), 121– 127.

Hanashiro, P. (1990). Hyperventilation: Benign symptom or harbinger of catastrophe? *Postgrad Med*, 88(1), 191– 196.

Harvey, S., Wood, D., & Feroah, T. (1997). Relationship of the head impulse test and head-shake nystagmus in reference to caloric testing. *Am J Otol*, 18, 207– 213.

Herdman, S., Tusa, R. J., Blatt, P., Suzuki, A., Venuto, P.J., & Roberts, D. (1998). Computerized dynamic visual acuity test in the assessment of vestibular deficits. *Am J Otol*, 19, 790– 796.

Hornsveld, H., & Garssen, B. (1996). The low specificity of the hyperventilation provocation test. *J Psychosom Res*, 41(5), 435– 449.

Hornsveld, H., Garssen, B., Dop, M. F., & Van Speigel, P. (1990). Symptom reporting during voluntary hyperventilation and mental load: Implications for diagnosing hyperventilation syndrome. *J Psychosom Res*, 34(6), 687– 697.

Jacob, R. G. (1988). Panic disorder and the vestibular system. *Psychiatr Clin North Am*, 11(2), 361– 374.

Jacobson, G., Newman, C., & Safadi, I. (1990). Sensitivity and specificity of the head-shaking test for detecting vestibular system abnormalities. *Ann Otol Rhinol Laryngol*, 90, 539– 542.

Kroenke, K., Lucas, C. A., Rosenberg, M. L., Sherokman, B., Herbers, J. E., Wehrle, P. A., et al. (1992). Causes of persistent dizziness: a prospective study of 100 patients in ambulatory care. *Ann Intern Med*, 117(11), 898– 905.

Leigh, R. J., & Zee, D. S. (1991). *The neurology of eye movements*, 2nd ed. Philadelphia: F.A. Davis.

Lempert, T., & Tiel-Wick, K. (1996). Positional maneuver for treatment of horizontal-canal benign positional vertigo. *Laryngoscope*, 106, 476– 478.

Linstrom, C. (1992). Office management of the dizzy patient. *Otolaryngol Clin North Am*, 25(4), 745– 780.

Longridge, N. S., & Mallinson, A. I. (1987). The dynamic illegible E (DIE) test: a simple technique for assessing the ability of the vestibulo-ocular reflex to overcome vestibular pathology. *J Otolaryngol*, *16*, 97–103.

Nozawa, I., Imamura, S., Hisamatsu, K., & Murakami, Y. (1996). The relationship between orthostatic dysregulation and the orthostatic test in dizzy patients. *Eur Arch Otorhinolaryngol*, *253*, 268–272.

Puisieux, F., Boumbar, Y., Bulckaen, H., Bonnin, E., Houssin, F., & Dewailly, P. (1999). Intraindividual variability in orthostatic blood pressure changes among older adults: The influence of meals. *J Am Geriatr Soc*, *47*, 1332–1336.

Sama, A., Meikle, J. C. E., & Jones, N. S. (1995). Hyperventilation and dizziness: case reports and management. *Br J Clin Pract*, *49*(2), 79–82.

Shepard, N. (1999). Integrated management of the balance disorder patient. In: *Vestibular update* (pp. 1–4). Vol 22. Chatham, IL: Micromedical Technologies.

Skiendzielewski, J. J., & Martyak, G. (1980). The weak and dizzy patient. *Ann Emerg Med*, *9*, 353–356.

Smith, D. (1991). Dizziness: A clinical perspective. In: *Vestibular update* (pp. 1–7). Vol 7. Chatham, IL: Micromedical Technologies.

Stark, R. J., & Wodak, J. (1983). Primary orthostatic cerebral ischaemia. *J Neurol Neurosurg Psychiatry*, *46*, 883–891.

Urbscheit, N. L., & Oremland, B. S. (1995). Cerebellar dysfunction. In: D.A. Umphred (Ed.), *Neurologic rehabilitation* (pp. 657–680). St. Louis: Mosby-Year Book.

Vansteenkiste, J., Rochette, F., & Demedts, M. (1991). Diagnostic tests of hyperventilation syndrome. *Eur Respir J*, *4*, 393–399.

Wollner, L., McCarthy, S. T., Soper, N. D. W., & Macy, D. J. (1979). Failure of cerebral auto-regulation as a cause of brain dysfunction in the elderly. *BMJ*, *1*, 1117–1118.

Zee, D. S., Fletcher, W. A. (1996). Bedside examination. In: R. W. Baloh, & C. M. Halmagyi (Eds.), *Disorders of the vestibular system* (pp. 178–190). New York: Oxford University Press.

4

Establishing and Equipping the Balance Clinic

A thorough history and physical examination will be sufficient to obtain a working diagnosis for many patients. When the history and initial examination do not provide sufficient information, electrophysiologic tests of the vestibular ocular reflex (VOR), screening for cerebellar dysfunction, or evaluation of postural stability may be indicated.

Traditionally, vestibular specialty clinics have been restricted to major teaching hospitals associated with a large university or medical school. This is largely because of the sizable obstacle of the cost of equipment encountered when considering adding vestibular evaluation capabilities to a clinic. The standard triad of vestibular evaluation equipment includes computerized electronystagmography (ENG), rotary chair testing, and computerized dynamic platform posturography. The cost of this equipment can approach, or even exceed, $200,000, which may prove cost prohibitive for many smaller private clinics. In the past several years, however, equipment manufacturers have been working to provide lower-cost alternatives in the attempt to allow more health care providers (HCPs) to focus on vestibular patients, thereby increasing access to appropriate care.

Electronystagmography or Videonystagmography Equipment

Videonystagmography (VNG), or ENG, is the most common method of vestibular evaluation (Bhansali & Honrubia, 1999). The advantages of ENG/ VNG over other vestibular tests include the ability to (1) document nystagmus for analysis; (2) examine cerebellar modulated voluntary eye movements, and (3) test one labyrinth at a time, which helps to localize the side of the lesion.

Limitations of ENG/VNG include (1) the inability to record (except visually) torsional or rotary eye movements common in benign paroxysmal positional vertigo (BPPV)[1]; (2) the lack of a wide-range stimulus in caloric testing (7°C above or below body temperature is a *very*-low-frequency stimulus): (3) evaluation of the horizontal canal only through caloric testing; (4) minimal information about the patient's level of central compensation; and (5) no information about the patient's functional abilities. A normal ENG/VNG examination cannot be interpreted as normal vestibular function.

Infrared Video Versus Electro-oculography

The term *electronystagmography* (electrical graph of nystagmus) has been used to describe a series of tests using *electro-oculography* (EOG), which refers to the recording of the electrical potentials associated with eye movements. The principle behind EOG is the recording of changes in the corneoretinal potential through the use of surface electrodes placed around the eyes. Electrodes placed at the outer canthi will record horizontal eye movement, and electrodes placed above and below the eye will record vertical eye movement. A reference electrode is placed farther away from the eyes.

The corneoretinal potential is the difference in electrical potential between the cornea (front of the eye: positively charged potential), and the retina (back of the eye: negatively charged potential). When the eye is moved to the right (Fig. 4–1A), there is an increase in the potential noted in the electrode beside the right eye and a decrease in potential in the electrode beside the left eye. This occurs simply because the positively charged cornea is closer to the right electrode and farther from the left electrode.

Infrared VOG (as used in VNG) involves the use of a conventional black and white video camera; however, the eyes are illuminated with infrared light. Because the eyes are not reactive to infrared light, the eye can be viewed while the patient's eyes are in total darkness, eliminating the possibility of visual

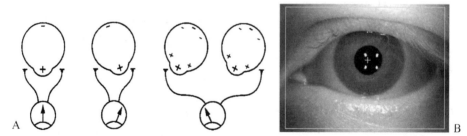

A   B

Figure 4–1. (A) Electro-oculography recording: The corneoretinal potential changes with eye movement and allows for accurate recording and measurement of eye movements. (B) Infrared video recording: Eye movement is recorded by tracking the dark part of the pupil

---

[1]Recently, a technique for recording rotary eye movements has been introduced which involves the recording of patterns on the iris, and allows measurement of any angle variation from baseline.

fixation, which is known to suppress peripheral vestibular-generated nystagmus. The camera is able to take rapid, sequential pictures of the eye, so even very fast eye movement can be recorded accurately. Because the picture is black and white, the eye is represented by black, white, and gray dots (or pixels). The pupil is a hole in the front of the eye that allows light to pass into the eye. As a result, it is not as reflective as the iris (the eye color portion) or the sclera (the "white" of the eye). Because the infrared light is not reflected from the pupil, it appears as a black spot on the screen (Fig. 4–1B), and this "dark spot" can be tracked for recording. A caveat of infrared recording is the fact that it will track the darkest spot in the camera's field. Dark-colored mascara, as well as the sides of the camera goggles, can sometimes be darker than the pupil. These problems can be overcome by removing mascara, adjusting the recording threshold of the computer, or packing white gauze into the sides of the goggles.

Several factors must be considered when making the decision to purchase ENG equipment. Significant differences exist between infrared video and EOG systems in the following areas: calibration, artifact, recording of rotary nystagmus, the presence of Bell's phenomenon, and cost-effectiveness. Each of these is discussed in detail in the following pages.

Potential Calibration Errors

The corneoretinal potential varies in response to the amount of light exposure, increasing with more light, decreasing in the dark. After exposure to light, an adaptation period follows that can last a few minutes or up to as long as 50 minutes. Norman and Brown (1999) showed a "marked shift" of about 20 to 30% in the amplitude of recordings over a 10-minute period following a change in room lighting. Hickson (1983) reported a 19% increase in trace amplitude following a 10-second exposure to light following adequate adaptation to dark. An analogous situation may be the speed of pupillary reaction to changes in lighting. We know that pupillary reaction is slower in the older population (Tiedeksar, 1989), and so it is possible that older patients will require additional time to adapt to lighting changes during vestibular testing.

Infrared video can record in any ambient lighting condition as well as in complete darkness. Because no adaptation period is required, testing can begin immediately on placement of the goggles, and introduction of light into the test room will not require recalibration. Recalibration is needed when the infrared camera is moved or repositioned.

Artifact

Electro-oculography is subject to contamination from ambient muscle electrical activity and artifact associated with eye blinks (Fig. 4–2). Eye blinks can occur with the eyes open or closed. Many patients exhibit activity in the vertical channel while their eyes are closed. Because this can be mistaken for vertical nystagmus, the eyes should be inspected visually for any type of eyelid flutter while the recording is taking place. Some older ENG equipment does not allow recordings in the vertical channel. The examiner must also be careful to rule out

Comparison of VNG and ENG Tracings

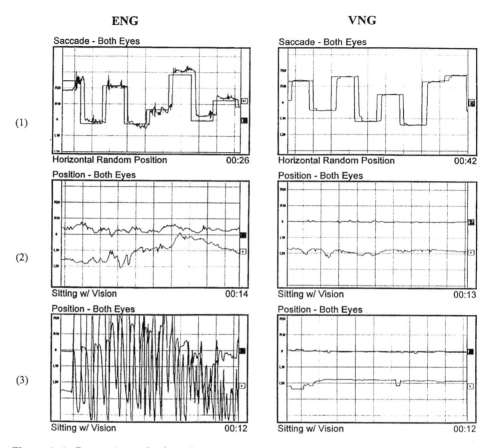

Figure 4–2. Comparison of infrared video (VNG) and electro-oculography (ENG) tracings: (1) Gritting teeth, jaw movement; (2) gritting teeth, jaw movement; (3) excessive eye blinks. The tracing on the left side of this figure shows excessive artifact from muscle activity and eye blinks. The tracings on the right show only the movement of the eye and do not record ambient muscle activity. (Reprinted with permission from ICS Medical promotional literature [undated]).

eye blinks or eyelid flutter, which also can be mistaken for horizontal nystagmus. Again, visual observation of the eyes eliminates misinterpretation of the recording. Even with VNG, eye blinks are visible on most recordings and inevitable temporary loss of tracking appears as artifact on the recording.

Recording of Rotary Nystagmus

The most common vestibular pathology is BPPV of the posterior semicircular canal. The nystagmus associated with this condition is torsional, moving in a clockwise or counterclockwise fashion. EOG recordings are possible only in the axis between two electrodes, which are placed vertically or horizontally to the eyes. Torsional nystagmus can be missed through EOG recordings, so it is imperative that the eyes be visualized during testing for BPPV. Stockwell (1996) advocates the use of Frenzel lenses or infrared video because the nystagmus associated with BPPV can be suppressed through visual fixation when the eyes are open (Stockwell, 1996), but the typical response is robust enough that it can easily be visualized with eyes open (Epley, 1994). The chances of misinterpretation are greater if the eyes remain closed. The use of Frenzel lenses or infrared video allows visualization of the eyes without introducing the possible artifact of visual fixation. It should be noted that the most current commercially available infrared video system also does not measure pure rotary or torsional eye movements for analysis. The interpretation of nystagmus associated with BPPV of the posterior canal is done through direct visual observation of the nystagmus. Horizontal nystagmus associated with BPPV of the horizontal canal is easily recorded through either technique.

Bell's Phenomenon

Bell's phenomenon refers to the rolling of the eyes superiorly and distally when the eyes are closed. This phenomenon can be seen when performing EOG-based ENG. When the patients close their eyes, the tracing must be recentered. This represents the eye rolling away from center with eyelid closure. Waldorf (1993) reports that, "In a few cases, patients who were tested with electrode ENG methods had abnormal or non-existent caloric responses. When their eyes were open in the IR/(infrared) video goggle, the nystagmic response became readily evident and recorded by the electrodes. Thus, the eyes open without fixation is an important advantage of the IR/Video ENG System." Goebel, Stroud, Levine, and Muntz (1983) reported that most patients could inhibit vestibular-induced (by calorics) nystagmus through vertical eye movement seen in Bell's phenomenon, but mental tasking proved effective in reducing or avoiding this inhibition.

Cost-Effectiveness

Infrared video recordings offer several advantages in terms of patient flow and cost effectiveness. The most obvious is the reduction in time needed to complete an ENG examination. In our office, an average of about 60 minutes is required per patient with EOG-based ENG and 45 to 50 minutes per patient with infrared video.

Another benefit of infrared video is that during the initial physical examination a quick screening for obvious spontaneous, gaze, or positional nystagmus is typically performed. Based on current Medicare reimbursement policies (which are subject to change), inspection for gaze or spontaneous or positional nystagmus is not reimbursable unless it is accompanied by a hard-copy recording. By performing this examination through infrared goggles with recording capabilities, the provider can be reimbursed. Of course, EOG-based recordings are also reimbursed, but the HCP must take the time to perform skin preparation, apply electrodes, and allow darkness adaptation time. Specific billing codes are discussed in Chapter 8. Infrared video does not require the use of electrodes, which provides cost savings of a few dollars per test.

The most notable disadvantage to infrared video is the fact that patients must keep their eyes open. Older and medicated patients sometimes have difficulty keeping their eyes open while in total darkness or when vertigo is induced. Patients who have small eyes or poor contrast between the pupil and the iris and sclera are better suited for EOG recordings. Some commercially available infrared systems offer the option of EOG recording capabilities, which can be used on an as-needed basis.

Computerized versus Strip-Chart Recordings

The two basic categories to consider when comparing conventional strip-chart recording with computerized analysis and recording systems are (1) tests that are easier to use with computerized programs, and (2) tests that are more accurate using computerized programs. There are no negatives associated with upgrading to computerized analysis hardware and software. The associated costs are quickly made up in savings of time.

Recording and measurement of horizontal and vertical nystagmus can be done accurately through strip-chart recording. Historically, the analysis involved considerable time in cutting and pasting (literally) samples of the paper tracing. Measurement of nystagmus was performed using a pencil and ruler and physically measuring the angle of the slope of the slow phase of individual nystagmus beats. Computerized ENG software allows measurement of the slow-phase velocity of individual beats as the testing is taking place. Artifacts are automatically rejected from analysis and the peak nystagmus response can be retrieved at the touch of the keypad.

Computerized generation of light bar stimulus and analysis of the recording benefit from much greater accuracy in the oculomotor portion of the ENG examination. Because the stimulus is computer controlled, many more aspects of eye movement can be accurately recorded. With strip-chart recordings, saccadic accuracy could be reasonably analyzed as long as the calibration was correct. Saccadic latency and velocity could not be measured accurately. Not only are the recordings more accurate, but the results can be compared with statistical norms for the patient's age and sex (Bhansali & Honrubia, 1999; Goebel 1992).

Because there are such significant benefits to computerized recording and data analysis, the major manufacturers of ENG/VNG equipment no longer offer new strip-chart systems. There are, however, still some strip charts in clinical use.

Caloric Irrigators

The caloric test is the most important part of the ENG examination (Bhansali & Honrubia, 1999) because it helps to lateralize vestibular pathology. The purpose of the caloric test is to determine the presence and degree of nystagmus response for cross comparison. It is performed by creating a temperature difference between the two labyrinths. Temperature change causes a change in density of the endolymph, and when the patient is appropriately positioned, will stimulate the horizontal semicircular canal. Warm stimulation results in an excitatory response, whereas cool stimulation results in an inhibitory response on the stimulated side (described in detail in Chapter 5).

The method of creating this temperature change has been a subject of much research, debate, and disagreement. Caloric stimulation may be accomplished by three different methods. Each has been scrutinized with no clear winner as to the preferred technique.

Open-loop water irrigation involves the direct introduction of water into the ear canal and is the predominant method of caloric stimulation (Karlsen, Mikhail, Norris, & Hassanein, 1992) (Fig. 4–3). This technique was first described by Robert Barany (Barany, 1916), and a standardized protocol was established by Fitzgerald and Hallpike (1942). Caloric test protocol is discussed in Chapter 5.

Closed-loop caloric irrigation involves using a latex balloon with heated water circulating through the balloon, allowing the ear canal to remain dry during stimulation (Fig. 4–4). This technique was introduced by Brookler, Baker, and Grams (1979) and became commercially available as the Brookler-Grams closed-loop system.

Air caloric stimulation involves the introduction of heated air into the ear canal (Fig. 4–5). Air is delivered from a pump, through an electrical heater, and then through a hose with a speculum placed in the ear canal.

Most clinicians prefer open-loop water irrigation because it has been demonstrated to induce the most robust response (Karlsen et al., 1992). Anderson (1995) reports that "A larger, stronger response is desirable when response measurement is inherently inaccurate if the response is weak. On the other hand, a large caloric response may well trigger autonomic reactions and considerable patient discomfort that may terminate the session prematurely, before clinically useful results have been obtained. The strongest response, therefore, may not be the most desirable aim."

The most notable limitation of open-water irrigation is the fact that it cannot be performed on patients with tympanic membrane perforations or pressure-equalization tubes. Closed-loop and air irrigations are safe with these patients.

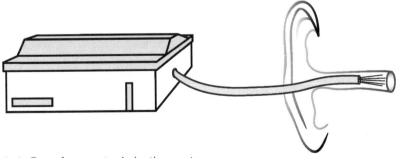

Figure 4–3. Open-loop water irrigation system.

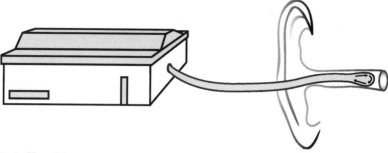

Figure 4–4. Closed-loop water irrigation system.

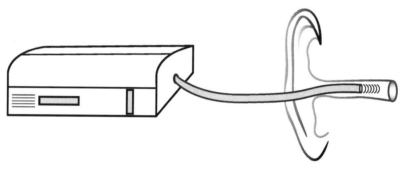

Figure 4–5. Air caloric irrigation system.

Barber, Harmand, and Money (1978), however, report that using air irrigation in a patient with a tympanic membrane perforation can result in nystagmus response opposite of that expected from warm air irrigation. Theoretically, the warm air evaporates the moisture in the middle ear cavity, causing a cooling effect, leading to an inhibitory rather than an excitatory response on the irrigated side.

Several investigators have noted that test–retest reliability is better with open-loop irrigations than with the other techniques (Henry, 1999; Zangemeister & Bock, 1979, 1980), whereas others have noted no significant difference (Ford & Stockwell, 1978; Karlsen et al., 1992; Munro & Higson, 1996; Suter, Blanchard, & Cook-Manokey, 1977; Tole, 1979; Westhofen, 1987). The closed-loop balloon method has been reported to be more comfortable for patients (Karlsen et al. 1992; Westhofen, 1987). Anderson (1995) describes maintenance and ease of use issues with each technique. He points out that open-water and air irrigators can typically be used with curved narrow ear canals, whereas the closed-loop balloon may be too flexible to navigate down the ear canal. Closed-loop and air irrigation systems are generally easier to operate because there is no water spillage. Air irrigators require minimal "warm-up" time compared with both water irrigators.

Other than routine maintenance, no ongoing costs are associated with air irrigators. Closed-loop irrigators require replacement balloons for each patient, and open-water irrigators require daily replenishment of sterile distilled water. The cost of the water is inconsequential compared with the time and effort required to keep a busy clinic stocked with heavy and space consuming bottles of water.

Manufacturers of ENG equipment (with their Web addresses) include the following:

Eye Dynamics (www.eyedynamics.com)
GN Otometrics (www.GNOtometrics.com)
AKA: ICS Medical (www.icsmedical.com)
Interacoustics (www.interacoustics.dk)
Micromedical Technologies (www.micromedical.com)
Senso Motoric Instruments (www.SMI.de)
Synapsys (www.synapsys.fr)

Rotational Test Equipment

Rotational testing provides information about the current state of the VOR, and results will typically change as central compensation occurs. Rotary tests can be performed using a rotary chair or through the use of an active head rotation (AHR) unit. Both units measure *gain* (amount of eye movement relative to head movement), *phase* (reaction time of the eyes in response to head movement), and *symmetry* (gain to rightward movement versus gain to leftward movement during sinusoidal head movement).

Rotational chair testing is considered "passive" rotation because the patient sits in a chair that is rotated by a servo-controlled torque motor (Fig. 4–6). The speed and velocity of rotation are controlled by the examiner and measured by a tachometer attached to the chair. The patient's head is restrained, so the assumption is made that chair speed and velocity equal head speed and velocity. The patient's eye movement responses are recorded through EOG or infrared video. Calculations of gain, phase, and symmetry can then be completed.

Rotary Chair versus Electronystagmography

Advantages of rotary chair testing over ENG include the use of a physiologic stimulus that can be performed at a number of frequencies. Caloric stimulation is aphysiologic and the stimulus creates a vestibular response that is analogous to an extremely slow head movement, below the range at which the VOR typically functions. Shepard and Telian (1996) report on a group of 2266 patients undergoing vestibular evaluation. Sixteen percent of these patients had completely normal ENG examinations. They report, "Among those with normal ENG results, rotary chair testing indicated abnormalities suggesting peripheral system pathology in 80% of cases, 35% by phase abnormalities and 45% by asymmetry findings."

Rotary chair testing is also better tolerated by patients, allowing serial examinations to document central compensation of peripheral vestibular injuries. Caloric testing is well tolerated by most patients but can lead to nausea and

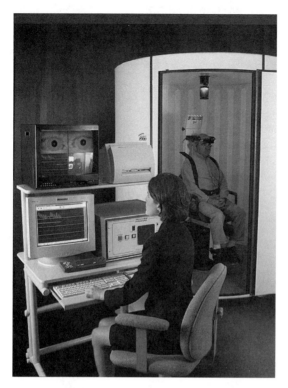

Figure 4–6. Typical rotational chair apparatus: Some newer systems do not require an enclosure because total darkness is achieved by having the patient wear goggles with infrared cameras. (Photo courtesy of Micromedical Technologies.)

vomiting on occasion. Repeat caloric testing will not reflect central compensation because caloric asymmetry resulting from vestibular injury is usually stable unless there has been a change in the function of the labyrinth. The primary disadvantage of rotary testing compared with caloric testing is that rotation stimulates both labyrinths, so lateralizing information is difficult to obtain.

Active Head Rotation

Active head rotation is considered "active" rotation because volitional movement on the part of the patient provides the rotary stimulus. The patient is asked to shake his or her head back and forth in the yaw and pitch planes. For patients having difficulty performing rapid, repetitive head shaking movements, the examiner can assist by manually rotating the patient's head with minimal effect on the results (Furman & Durrant, 1998). The apparatus used in AHR involves a motion sensor attached to a head-worn band or goggles, strapped tightly to minimize slippage (Fig. 4–7). The motion sensor measures head speed and velocity; EOG or infrared video recordings of eye movements are completed simultaneously. Patients are instructed to shake their head in a sinusoidal fashion, keeping time with a computer-generated audible tone. The same calculations of gain, phase, and symmetry are performed.

Active Head Rotation versus Electronystagmography

Active head rotation testing has been shown to be significantly more sensitive than ENG in detecting abnormalities in patients with reports of balance disorders. Saddat, O'Leary, Pulec, and Kitano (1995) performed both caloric testing and AHR on 39 patients complaining of balance disorders. Of this group,

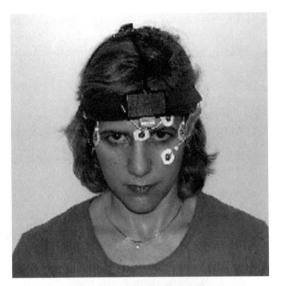

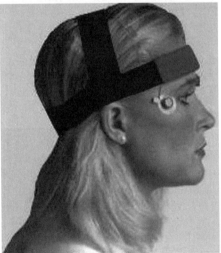

Figure 4–7. Active head rotation system: Specifically, the vestibular autorotation system (VAT) by Western Systems Research. (Reprinted from O'Leary, D. P., Davis, L. L., & Kevorkian, K. F. (1990). Dynamic analysis of age-related responses of the vestibulo-ocular reflex. In: L. O'Leary. (Ed.). *The VAT for testing balance* (pp. 194– 202). (Photo courtesy of Western Systems Research, Pasadena, CA).

24 had abnormal caloric studies, but 37 had abnormal AHR tests. In the same study, they found that 4 of 10 patients with confirmed acoustic neuroma had normal caloric studies, but all 10 had abnormal AHR tests. In contrast, bilaterally absent caloric responses might be misinterpreted as an absence of vestibular function if higher frequency rotational tests are not performed. Goebel and Rowden (1992) report that two thirds of a group of 34 patients exhibiting bilaterally reduced caloric responses had normal gain of the VOR at 0.5 Hz. This type of information is critical to designing a customized vestibular rehabilitation program because the therapy for patients with total loss of vestibular function differs from those with residual vestibular function. Caloric testing only stimulates the horizontal semicircular canal, whereas AHR records the response to horizontal *and* vertical head movement, allowing evaluation of the VOR in more than one plane.

Most vestibular specialists agree that ENG alone is insufficient to evaluate many patients with vestibular dysfunction and that some type of rotational testing is an important component of the test battery of a balance clinic. There is more disagreement as to whether rotational chair or AHR provides more useful information.

Rotary Chair versus Active Head Rotation

The main clinical difference between rotary chair tests and AHR is the speed at which the VOR is being tested. Rotary chair tests the response of the VOR to relatively slow movement, which may be more sensitive to progressive vestibular lesions. Insufficient torque to drive the chair and uncontrolled head slippage limit the chair's ability to test moderate to rapid speed head movements accurately. Hanson and Goebel (1995) report that rotary chair testing provides a reliable measure of VOR gain and phase at speeds below 0.5 Hz using standard head restraint techniques. Between 0.5 Hz and 1.0 Hz, additional head restraint allows for reliable testing. Above 1 Hz, head movement cannot be controlled adequately and rotary chair testing becomes unreliable. Because of this, rotary chair tests traditionally do not test frequencies above 1.0 Hz. Natural head movements typically occur at higher speeds, and so the functional importance of VOR gain and phase at less than 1.0 Hz is questionable (Hirvonen, Aalto, Pyykko, & Jantti, 1997).

Active head rotation measures faster, more real-life frequencies of head movement and simulates the condition (rapid head movement) most likely to elicit a complaint from a patient with vestibular dysfunction. The primary role of the VOR is to stabilize the eyes relative to the environment while the head is moving, allowing for clear vision. It does this by causing eye movements that are equal and opposite to head movements. Head movements in daily life typically occur between 0.5 and 5.0 Hz; however, the VOR can respond efficiently up to 8 Hz (Gresty, Hess, & Leech, 1977; Sawyer et al. 1994). Cerebellar-controlled voluntary eye movements function efficiently up to around 1.0 Hz and can contribute to clear vision during slower head movement, even in the absence of vestibular function. Above 2.0 Hz, only the VOR can contribute to gaze stability.

Head slippage of the motion sensor is less of an issue because of the decreased mass of the smaller AHR unit. Additionally, an algorithm to offset head slippage from calculations of gain and phase has been developed. Some researchers advocate the use of a "bite board" to hold the motion sensor firmly but recognize that this may be difficult to implement in the clinic (Meulenbroeks, Kingma, van Twisk, & Vermeulen, 1995). The influence of the cervico-ocular reflex (COR) on AHR has been noted as a potential disadvantage of AHR. The COR is negligible in patients with normal vestibular function, and the contribution of the COR to gaze stability in the absence of vestibular function has been recorded only at very low frequencies (0.5 Hz) (Barlow & Freedman, 1980; Kasai & Zee, 1978). Another noted disadvantage of AHR is the fact that many patients cannot perform rapid head movements required for a full range of testing (Guyot & Psillas, 1997). In contrast, Furman, and Durrant (1998) report that even older patients were able to consistently produce head movements up to 3 Hz. Hirvonen, Pyykko, Aalto, and Juhola (1997) suggest that, in patients of working age, the inability to reach a head rotation speed of 4.0 Hz may indicate an abnormality of the vestibular system.

Both techniques reliably evaluate the compensated state of the VOR for a particular frequency range. Comparative studies have shown good agreement between rotary chair and AHR in the mid frequencies. (Goebel, Isipradit, & Hanson, 2000) The results of rotary chair and AHR cannot be compared because they test different aspects of the vestibular response. A patient may have normal AHR and abnormal rotary chair or vice versa. One cannot predict the outcome of one rotary test (AHR or rotary chair) based on the outcome of the other. The ideal situation would allow VOR testing for the full range of frequencies, from as low as that evaluated by ENG (.003 Hz) to as high as can be generated by the patient (typically 3.0 to 6.0 Hz).

Other factors to consider when deciding between rotary chair and AHR is the sizable difference in cost of equipment, time to perform the test, and space requirements. Rotary chair has the advantage of being considered the "gold standard," has been the subject of much research, and is generally considered to have better test–retest reliability than AHR (Henry & DiBartolomeo, 1993). On the negative side, rotary chair costs are in range of $50,000 to $100,000 and require a dedicated space of approximately 10 by 10 feet. Active head rotation systems can be purchased for less than $20,000 (much less when purchased along with a computerized ENG system) and require no additional dedicated space. AHR can be performed in the same room as the ENG, using the same light bar for the target. AHR also typically can be completed in much less time than rotary chair testing of several frequencies. Some vestibular specialists consider AHR experimental and are critical of its test–retest reliability (Guyot & Psillas, 1997). In my opinion, AHR serves an important adjunctive role but is not a substitute for rotational chair testing.

Manufacturers of rotational chair and AHR equipment include the following:

>GN Otometrics (www.GNOtometrics.com)
>AKA: ICS Medical (www.icsmedical.com)
>Micromedical Technologies – VORTEQ (www.micromedical.com)

Western Systems Research – Vestibular Autorotation Test (VAT)
(www.4wsr.com)

POSTUROGRAPHY EQUIPMENT

Postural stability assessment can be performed with minimal equipment. Using some type of computerized force plate that measures center of gravity and sway, however, provides numeric data, which can be compared with the established norms or used to document outcome. Unlike other vestibular tests, posturo-graphy is not a test of the VOR. Standard tests of the VOR evaluate the response of the horizontal semicircular canal but provide no information about the otolith structures or the vestibular spinal reflex (VSR). Some researcher have suggested that posturography is a test of VSR function, but this has been disputed by others (Asai, Watanabe, Ojashi, & Mizukoshi, 1993; Black & Wall, 1981; Evans & Krebs, 1999). The most useful form of posturography in the evaluation of vestibular patients is the sensory organization test (SOT), which involves measuring the patient's response to a variety of visual and somatosensory altered conditions. Depending on the equipment used, SOT can involve four or six sensory conditions. Although there are slight variations in how the six conditions are accomplished, they follow a standard pattern of progressively reducing or distorting information used for the maintenance of balance. As the conditions become progressively more difficult, the patient is forced to rely more on visual, somatosensory, or vestibular inputs individually.

The following are the six conditions:

Condition One: Stable platform with eyes open in a stable visual environment (patient has full use of all information—visual, vestibular, and somatosensory)
Condition Two: Stable platform with eye closed (patient must rely on vestibular and somatosensory information)
Condition Three: Stable platform with moving visual surround (patient must suppress a false sense of visually induced movement and rely on vestibular and somatosensory inputs)
Condition Four: Unstable platform with eyes open in a stable visual environment (patient must rely on vestibular and visual inputs)
Condition Five: Unstable platform with eyes closed (patient must rely primarily on vestibular input as visual and somatosensory feedback have been eliminated)
Condition Six: Unstable platform and unstable visual environment (patient must rely primarily on vestibular input and suppress a false sense of visually induced movement)

These six conditions can be accomplished in a number of ways. The "gold standard" of posturography is computerized dynamic posturography (CDP) using the Equitest produced by NeuroCom International (Fig. 4–8). This test has been the subject of much research regarding its clinical value, sensitivity, and specificity in identifying patients with vestibular disorders. The Equitest produces an unstable visual surround by causing the wall in front of the patient to move in response to the patient's sway as measured on the base platform. When the patient leans forward, the wall moves forward synchronously, therefore distorting visual feedback of movement. Reduced somatosensory feedback is accomplished by movement of the base platform in response to the patient's sway. When the patient leans forward, the platform moves as well, therefore reducing or distorting proprioceptive feedback normally received from the stretch receptors of the lower legs (Fig. 4–9). The cost of the Equitest is around $80,000.

Informal SOT was described by Shumway-Cook and Horak (1986) and is referred to as the clinical test of sensory integration and balance (CTSIB). This technique is also known as "foam and dome" because alterations in somatosensory and visual feedback are accomplished by having the patient stand on a foam surface or wearing a Chinese lantern over his or her head (Fig. 4–10).

NeuroCom has introduced a lower cost posturography unit that allows for limited sensory organization testing. The Balance Master ($13,000 to $25,000) is a spring-loaded platform that measures sway and center of gravity. The software program includes a SOT that uses only four conditions. These conditions are similar in effect to conditions one, two, four, and five as described previously. Elimination of visual feedback is accomplished by having patients close their eyes. Reduction or distortion of somatosensory feedback is accomplished by having the patient stand on an 8-inch foam surface situated on top of the base platform. Conditions involving altered or distorted visual feedback are not assessed.

Micromedical Technologies has introduced a line of posturography equipment. They offer the Balance Check (cost $12,500), which allows the examiner to perform a modified CTSIB and to evaluate the limits of stability (LOS). The Balance Quest (cost $64,000) is their version of CDP. It differs from the Equitest in that different visual environments are provided through virtual-reality glasses; an optokinetic effect is produced through a mirror ball projecting moving visual scene on the wall surrounding the patient. The Balance Quest does not have a motor control test (MCT), described earlier as part of the Equitest protocol.

The SOT is not a diagnostic site of lesion test but rather provides information about the patient's functional abilities. Certain response patterns are associated with vestibular dysfunction; however, one cannot make the diagnosis of vestibular dysfunction based on posturographic information alone. These patterns are discussed in Chapter 5. SOT information is helpful in formulating a specific therapy plan for balance-disordered patients.

Manufacturers of posturography equipment include the following:

> NeuroCom International (www.onbalance.com)
> Micromedical Technologies (www.micromedical.com)

SENSORY ORGANIZATION PROTOCOL

Condition	Vision	Support	Patient Instructions
1 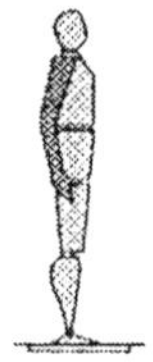	Normal	Fixed	Stand quietly with your eyes OPEN
2 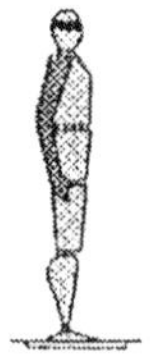	Absent	Fixed	Stand quietly with your eyes CLOSED
3 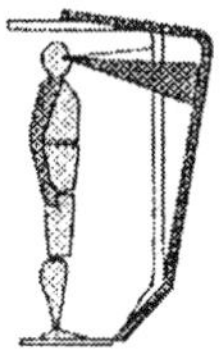	SwayRef	Fixed	Stand quietly with your eyes OPEN
4 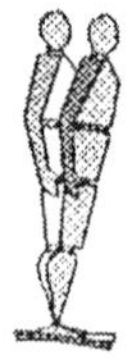	Normal	SwayRef	Stand quietly with your eyes OPEN
5 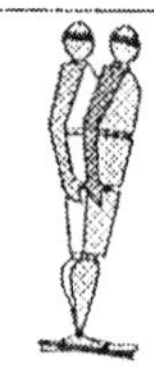	Absent	SwayRef	Stand quietly with your eyes CLOSED
6 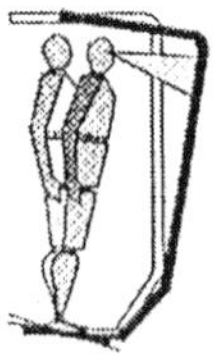	SwayRef	SwayRef	Stand quietly with your eyes OPEN

Figure 4–8. Six conditions of sensory organization testing as performed on the Equitest by NeuroCom. (Reprinted with permission from Shepard and Telian, 1996)

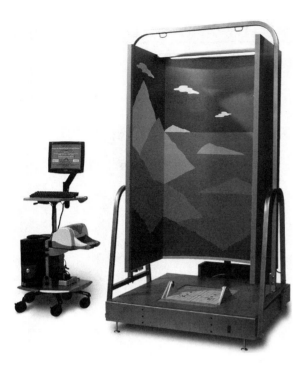

Figure 4–9. Equitest: by Neuro-Com International. (Photo courtesy of NeuroCom International.)

Frenzel Lenses

Frenzel lenses are used to examine the patient for nystagmus that may be suppressed by visual fixation (Fig. 4–11). Frenzel lenses are + 30-magnified lenses housed in a light-tight frame. Lights inside the frame illuminate the lenses, allowing magnification and illumination of the eyes while at the same time reducing the patient's vision to reduce visual fixation. Assessment of nystagmus should be performed in a darkened room because the patient may still be able to achieve some level of fixation in a lighted room (Baloh & Honrubia, 1990). Hain (1993) warns that although the distortion caused by Frenzel's lenses will reduce visual fixation, it may not have the same effect as total darkness achieved using infrared goggles, and comparisons of intensity of nystagmus should be viewed with caution.

Equipping the Vestibular Rehabilitation Facility

The equipment needed for performing vestibular rehabilitation (VR) is relatively inexpensive compared with the facilities required for most aspects of vestibular diagnostic testing. A larger room is preferable, but nearly all VR activities can be performed in a 10-by-10-ft space so long as there is a long, unobstructed hallway available. The therapy room should be equipped with a monitoring camera and videocassette recorder to record all therapy sessions. Exercise equipment can be

NORMAL   BLINDFOLD   DOME

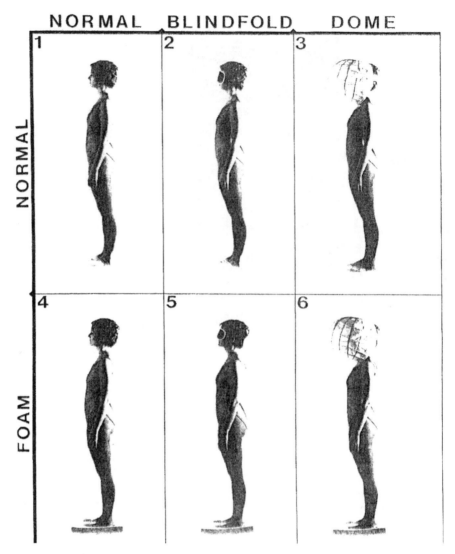

Figure 4–10. Foam and dome technique. (Reprinted with permission from Shumway-Cook, A., & Horak, F. (1986). Assessing the influence of sensory interaction on balance. *Phys Ther, 66*, 1548.)

purchased from a number of vendors (one supplier offers a "Vestibular Rehabilitation Kit"), or many of the needed items can be made by the therapist or purchased from a local department store. The exercises listed in Chapter 6 and described in Appendix C incorporate most of the equipment:

In the following list, which is incomplete but is representative of the types and costs of equipment that may be useful in performing VR therapy:

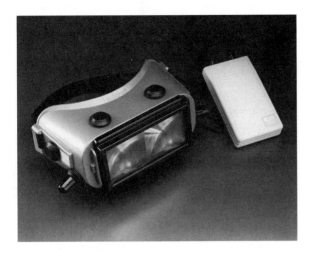

Figure 4–11. Frenzel lenses: The box houses batteries that provide power to the light source inside the goggles. (Photo courtesy of ICS Medical.)

Balance beam— for hip strategies exercises. $85 to $125

Large, thick foam mat (8 inches thick, 4 ft by 8 ft)— for compliant surface while walking and for patient safety. $115 to $230

Full-length lightweight movable wall mirror— to provide visual feedback. $250 to $370

Mini-trampoline— for compliant surface and vertical VOR stimulus. $60 to $140

Physioballs (large and small)— for hip strategy and vertical VOR exercises. $15 to $22

Lightweight 12-inch rubber ball— for ball toss and kick exercises. $1 to $2

Safety belt— to support patient during exercises. $25 to $35

Metronome— to time head and eye movements. $15 to $25

Kitchen timer— to time exercises. $1 to $5

Balance board— for hip strategy exercises. $75 to $150

Exam table— for Canalith repositioning procedures. $270 to $400

Balance Master— training software provides visual feedback for weight shifts. $13,000 to $25,000

Suppliers include the following:

Abilations, Select Service and Supply Co., Inc., One Sportime Way, Atlanta GA 30340

Smith & Nephew, Inc., One Quality Drive, P.O. Box 1005, Germantown, WI 53022-8205

Flaghouse, 150 North MacQueston Parkway, Mount Vernon, NY 10550

NeuroCom International (www.onbalance.com)

References

Anderson, S. (1995). Caloric irrigators: air, open-loop water and closed-loop water. *Br J Audiol*, *29*, 117–128.

Asai, M., Watanabe, Y., Ojashi, N., & Mizukoshi, K. (1993). Evaluation of vestibular function by dynamic posturography and other equilibrium examinations. *Acta Otolaryngol, 504*, 120–124.

Baloh, R. W., & Honrubia, V. (1990). *Clinical neurophysiology of the vestibular system*, 2nd ed. Philadelphia: F.A. Davis.

Barany, R. (1916). Some new methods for functional testing of the vestibular apparatus and the cerebellum. *Nobel lectures*, 1901–1921. Amsterdam-London-New York: Elsevier.

Barber, H., Harmand, W., & Money, K. (1978). Air caloric stimulation with tympanic membrane perforation. *Laryngoscope*, *88*, 1117–1126.

Barlow, D., & Freedman, W. (1980). Cervico-ocular reflex in the normal adult, *Acta Otolaryngol*, *89*, 487–496.

Bhansali, S., & Honrubia, V. (1999). Current status of electronystagmography testing. *Otolaryngol Head Neck Surg*, *120*(3), 419–426.

Black, F. O., & Wall, C. (1981). Comparison of vestibulo-ocular and vestibulospinal screening tests. *Otolaryngol Head Neck Surg*, 89, 811–817.

Brookler, K. H., Baker, A. H., & Grams, G. (1979). Closed loop water irrigation system. *Otolaryngol Head Neck Surg*, *87*, 364–365.

Epley, J. M. (1994). Fine points of the canalith repositioning procedure for treatment of BPPV. *Insights Otolaryngol*, *9*(2), 1–8.

Evans, M., & Krebs, D. (1999). Posturography does not test vestibulospinal function. *Otolaryngol Head Neck Surg*, *120*(2), 164–173.

Fitzgerald, H., & Hallpike, C. (1942). Studies in human vestibular function: Observations on the directional preponderance of caloric nystagmus, *Brain*, *65*, 115–137.

Ford, C. R., & Stockwell, C. W. (1978). Reliabilities of air and water caloric responses. *Arch Otolaryngol*, *104*(7), 380–382.

Furman, J., & Durrant, J. (1998). Head-only rotational testing in the elderly. *J Vestib Res*, *8*(5), 355–361.

Goebel, J. (1992). Contemporary diagnostic update: Clinical utility of computerized oculomotor and posture testing. *Am J Otol*, *13*(6), 591–597.

Goebel, J. A., Isipradit, P., & Hanson, J. M. (2000). Manual rotational testing of the vestibulo-ocular reflex. *Laryngoscope*, *110*(4), 517–535.

Goebel, J., & Rowdon, D. (1992). Utility of headshake versus whole-body VOR evaluation during routine electronystagmography. *Am J Otol*, *13*(3), 249–253.

Goebel, J. A., Stroud, M. H., Levine, L. A., & Muntz, H. R. (1983). Vertical eye deviation and nystagmus inhibition during mental tasking. *Laryngoscope*, *93*(9), 1127–1132.

Gresty, M. A., Hess, K., & Leech, J. (1977). Disorders of the vestibulo-ocular reflex producing oscillopsia and mechanisms compensating for loss of labyrinthine function. *Brain*, *100*, 693–716.

Guyot, J., & Psillas, G. (1997). Test–retest reliability of vestibular autorotation testing in healthy subjects. *Otolaryngol Head Neck Surg*, *117*(6), 704–707.

Hain, T. (1993). Background and technique of ocular motility testing. In: G. P. Jacobson, C. W. Newman, & J. M. Kartush (Eds.), *Handbook of balance function testing* (pp. 83–100). St. Louis: Mosby Year Book.

Hanson, J., & Goebel, J. (1995). Head slippage during broad-frequency rotational chair testing. *J Vestib Res*, *5*(5), 371–376.

Henry, D. (1999). Test–retest reliability of open-loop bithermal caloric irrigation responses from healthy young adults. *Am J Otol*, *20*, 220–222.

Henry, D. F., & Di Bartolomeo, J. D. (1993). Closed-loop caloric, harmonic acceleration and active head rotation tests: norms and reliability. *Otolaryngol Head Neck Surg.*, 109: 975–987.

Hickson, F. S. (1983). Illuminance and recording of eye movements by electro-oculography. *Br J Audiol*, *17*(1), 11–16.

Hirvonen, T., Aalto, H., Pyykko, I. J., & Jantti, P. (1997a). Changes in vestibulo-ocular reflex of elderly people. *Acta Otolaryngol*, *529*, 198–110.

Hirvonen, T., Pyykko, I., Aalto, H., & Juhola, M. (1997b). Vestibulo-ocular reflex function as measured with the head autorotation test. *Acta Otolaryngol*, *117*, 657–662.

Kasai, T., & Zee, D. (1978). Eye–head coordination in labyrinthe defective human beings. *Brain Res, 144*, 123–141.

Karlsen, E., Mikhail, H. H., Norris, C. W., & Hassanein, R. S. (1992). Comparison of responses to air, water, and closed-loop caloric irrigators. *J Speech Hear Res, 35*, 186–191.

Meulenbroeks, A. A. W. M., Kingma, H., Van Twisk, J. J., & Vermeulen, M. P. (1995). Quantitative evaluation of the vestibular autorotation test (VAT) in normal subjects. *Acta Otolaryngol, 520*, 327–333.

Munro, K.J., & Higson, J.M. (1996). The test–retest variability of the caloric test: a comparison of a modified air irrigation with the conventional water technique. *Br J Audiol, 30*(5), 303–306.

Norman, M., & Brown, E. (1999). Variations in calibration for computerized electronystagmography. *Br J Audiol, 33*, 1–7.

O'Leary, D. P., Davis, L. L., & Kevorkian, K. F. (1990). Dynamic analysis of age-related responses of the vestibulo-ocular reflex. In: L. O'Leary. (Ed.). *The VAT for testing balance* (pp. 194–202). Western Systems Research.

Saadat, D., O'Leary, D., Pulec, J., & Kitano, H. (1995). Comparison of vestibular autorotation and caloric testing. *Otolaryngol Head Neck Surg, 113*(3), 215–222.

Sawyer, R. N. Jr, Thurston, S. E., Becker, K. R., Ackley, C. V., Seidman, S. H., & Leigh, J. R. (1994). The cervico-ocular reflex of normal human subjects in response to transient and sinusoidal trunk rotation. *J Vestib Res, 4*(3), 245–249.

Shepard, N. T., & Telian, S. A. (1996). Practical management of the balance disorder patient. San Diego: Singular Publishing Group.

Shumway-Cook, A., & Horak, F. (1986). Assessing the influence of sensory interaction on balance. *Phys Ther, 66*, 1548.

Stockwell, C. (1996, May). Tutorial on the three forms of benign positional vertigo (BPV). *ICS Medical*, 1–5.

Suter, C. M., Blanchard, C. L., & Cook-Manokey, B. E. (1977). Nystagmus responses to water and air caloric stimulation in clinical populations. *Laryngoscope, 87*(7), 1074–1078.

Tideiksaar, R. (1989). Medical causes of falling. In: R. Tideiksaar (Ed.), *Falling in old age: Its prevention and treatment* (pp. 21–47). New York: Springer.

Tole, J. R. (1979). A protocol for the air caloric test and a comparison with a standard water caloric test. *Arch Otolaryngol, 105*(6), 314–319.

Waldorf, R. A. (1993). Observations of eye movements related to vestibular and other neurological problems using the House infrared/Video ENG system. In I. K. Arenberg (Ed.), *Dizziness and balance disorders: An interdisciplinary approach to diagnosis treatment and rehabilitation* (pp. 277–281). New York: Kugler.

Westhofen, M. (1987). Balloon method and water irrigation in thermal vestibular assessment. Electronystagmographic comparison of both methods. *Ann Laryngol Rhinol Otolaryngol, 66*(8), 424–427.

Zangemeister, W. H., & Bock, O. (1979). Air caloric test: as useful as the water caloric test. *Ann Laryngol Rhinol Otol, 58*(4), 323–327.

Zangemeister, W. H., & Bock, O. (1980). Air versus water caloric test. *Clin Otolaryngol, 5*(6), 379–387.

5

Vestibular Evaluation

When information obtained through examination of the case history and screening examinations described in Chapter 3 is insufficient to provide a diagnosis, additional evaluation of the vestibular ocular reflex (VOR), cerebellar function, and postural stability may be indicated. The evaluation of the balance-disordered patient has two specific goals: (1) locating the site of the lesion and (2) assessing the patient's functional ability. This involves a number of tests to evaluate different parts of the vestibular apparatus and neural structures involved in the maintenance of balance.

The patient's presenting complaints and outward signs help in determining which of the following tests are indicated. A complete evaluation of the systems consists of audiometric evaluation, electronystagmography (ENG), rotational tests of the VOR, posturographic studies, and auditory brain stem response (ABR). Norre (1994) advocates performing the full battery of tests before arriving at a diagnosis. He points out that "concerning the 'relevance' of history, it is obvious that one cannot rely upon history alone, as has been proposed." Norre (1994) goes further to state that "despite urging the patient to give a clear description, the history as such is not always reliable or indicative in the same degree for each patient. Regularly, an important number of patients present a rather imprecise and atypical history." He found that only two thirds of patients ultimately diagnosed with benign paroxysmal positional vertigo (BPPV) provided histories suggestive of the condition. Keim (1985) cautions against performing only vestibular evaluation based on patients with the specific complaints of vertigo and suggests that evaluation criteria be more inclusive.

Audiometric Evaluation

Audiometric evaluation is a necessary starting point for a number of reasons, but it primarily provides information about auditory asymmetry, possible retro-cochlear pathologies, and the health and integrity of the ear canal and tympanic membrane before caloric irrigation (Flickinger-Moorehead & Downs, 1993).

Audiometric evaluation consists of pure-tone air and bone-conduction thresholds; speech audiometry, including speech recognition threshold (SRT) and speech recognition tests; tympanometry; acoustic reflex threshold and decay tests; rollover tests; and, when indicated, otoacoustic emissions (OAEs) (see Glossary for definitions of each test).

Auditory Symmetry

Auditory asymmetry refers to a significant difference in hearing levels between the ears and indicates the possibility of peripheral vestibular or auditory nerve pathology. The Mayo Clinic (Robinette, Bauch, Olsen, & Cevette, 2000) uses a criterion of a "difference of 15 dB or greater averaged across 500, 1000, 2000, 3000 Hz or differences of 15 dB or greater in speech recognition thresholds" to determine *significant* asymmetry.

Although there are numerous causes for asymmetric auditory sensitivity, including middle ear pathologies, various patterns have been linked with specific vestibular disease. Endolymphatic hydrops (Meniere's disease) is frequently accompanied by unilateral, fluctuating, low-frequency sensorineural hearing loss (Andrews & Honrubia, 1996). Acoustic neuroma is often characterized by an asymmetry in the higher frequencies (NIH Consensus Statement, 1991). Perilymph fistula and labyrinthitis are usually accompanied by unilateral sensorineural hearing loss with no specific pattern or configuration of loss.

Retrocochlear Pathology

Retrocochlear pathology refers to site of lesion at the cranial nerve (CN) VIII, cerebellopontine angle, or root entry zone of the CN VIII into the brain stem. A number of audiometric findings are suggestive of retrocochlear site of lesion and may be found in acoustic neuroma, multiple sclerosis, and a variety of brain stem lesions (Flickinger-Moorehead & Downs, 1993). Audiometric signs consistent with possible retrocochlear pathology include the following:

1. Asymmetric, typically high-frequency, sensorineural hearing loss
2. Speech recognition scores[1] poorer than would be expected based on audiometric configuration and severity (NIH Consensus Statement, 1991)
3. Rollover[1] or decreased speech recognition scores with higher intensity speech presentation levels (Jerger & Jordan, 1980)
4. Absent or elevated acoustic reflex thresholds[1] or abnormal acoustic reflex decay (Silman, 1984).

The Ear Canal and Tympanic Membrane

The health and integrity of the ear canal and tympanic membrane must be ascertained before beginning vestibular evaluation. Many patients with middle ear pathology will complain of dizziness as well as other auditory symptoms. It is

[1]These terms are defined in the glossary.

prudent to treat the middle ear problem first to determine whether there is an improvement in the complaint of "dizziness." Also, treatment might remove confounding factors affecting sensitive evaluation, such as aural fullness, tinnitus, and otalgia, which are common to both middle ear and peripheral vestibular disorders. Conditions such as tympanic membrane perforation, cerumen impaction, external otitis, or discharge may contraindicate open-loop water caloric irrigation of the external auditory canal.

Special Audiometric Tests

AUDITORY-EVOKED POTENTIALS

Auditory-evoked potentials (AEPs) or ABR are used to determine the integrity of the auditory/vestibular nerve (CN VIII). Any vestibular asymmetry noted on rotational tests or caloric studies can involve lesions of CN VIII or the peripheral vestibular apparatus. The most common abnormality associated with abnormal AEPs (excepting hearing loss) is a cerebellopontine angle tumor, specifically a vestibular schwannoma. These are more commonly referred to as *acoustic neuroma*. Studies have shown this test to be highly sensitive in detecting acoustic neuroma (NIH Consensus Statement, 1991). AEP testing may not detect small acoustic tumors. Schmidt, Sataloff, Newman, Spiegel, and Myers (2001) report that AEP/ABR had only a 58% sensitivity in detecting tumors smaller than 1 cm; however, it has a 94% or better rate of sensitivity in tumors larger than 1 cm. Schmidt et al. (2001) also report that all patients in the "small" tumor group exhibited asymmetrical sensorineural hearing loss, and none described vestibular complaints.

Imaging studies are gradually replacing the ABR as the test of choice for suspected acoustic neuroma; however, the cost of magnetic resonance imaging (MRI) with contrast still makes ABR a viable and effective test (Robinette et al., 2000). In addition, a screening MRI scan may not detect demyelinating conditions, such as multiple sclerosis, in which case ABR tests are frequently abnormal if the condition is affecting the auditory/vestibular pathways to the brain (Robinette et al., 2000; Shelton, Harnsbarger, Allen, & King, 1996).

ELECTROCOCHLEOGRAPHY

Electrocochleography in vestibular evaluation is often used as an objective measure of possible endolymphatic hydrops (EH) associated with Meniere's disease. Patients with EH often have a recordable increase in endocochlear potentials, particularly the summating potential (SP). Electrocochleography involves measuring the amplitude of the SP as a ratio of the action potential (AP), which represents the response of CN VIII. Patients with active EH may have a higher SP:AP ratio than do patients with normal vestibular function. Depending on the recording techniques, the sensitivity of electrocochleography falls between 60 and 65%, higher if the patient is acutely symptomatic at the time of testing (Ferraro, 2000).

OTOACOUSTIC EMISSIONS

Otoacoustic emissions (OAEs) are sounds generated by a healthy cochlea, which can be recorded in the ear canal. In cases in which dizziness is associated with unilateral fluctuating or sudden-onset sensorineural hearing loss, OAEs can be helpful in separating cochlear from neural pathology. OAEs will be present if the hearing loss is a result of auditory nerve pathology such as acoustic neuroma or vestibular neuronitis, whereas they will be absent in the presence of cochlear pathology. An exception to this rule is the fact that OAEs may be present in patients with Meniere's disease, even in the presence of significant cochlear hearing loss (Ohlms, Lounsbery-Martin, & Martin, 1991). Administration of glycerol to Meniere's patients can increase temporarily the amplitude of OAEs as well as improve hearing thresholds and speech understanding (Martin, Ohlms, Franklin, Harris, & Lonsbury-Martin, 1990).

GLYCEROL TEST FOR ENDOLYMPHATIC HYDROPS

Dehydrating agents such as glycerol or urea can temporarily reverse the effects of EH. Theoretically, glycerol in the bloodstream dehydrates the inner ear, improving cochlear function and hearing (Yellin, Waller, & Roland, 1993). "Oral dosage of 1.2 ml (of glycerol)/kg of body weight with the addition of an equal amount of physiologic saline" is recommended by Lee, Paparella, Margolis, and Le (1995). Instructions to refrain from eating or drinking for at least 6 hours before arrival are given to the patient when scheduling the appointment. The patient undergoes baseline audiometry just before drinking the glycerol/saline solution and then undergoes hourly audiometric examinations for 3 hours after ingestion of the solution. A 10-dB improvement in two or more adjacent pure-tone thresholds and a 12% improvement in speech recognition ability are considered to be a positive glycerol test and highly diagnostic for EH. A subjective decrease in aural pressure and tinnitus may also be noted by the patient (Lee et al., 1995; Yellin et al., 1993). Glycerol testing has gradually been replaced by performing electrocochleography (discussed earlier in this chapter). Some clinics are not equipped to perform electrocochleography. Glycerol testing does not require equipment beyond that used for basic audiometric testing.

ELECTRONYSTAGMOGRAPHY

The eyes are the window to the vestibular system and not only provide information about peripheral vestibular function but also provide information regarding the ability to generate efficient voluntary eye movements necessary for maintaining visual contact with one's environment.

Electronystagmography (ENG) consists of three subtests or subgroupings of tests known as (1) oculomotor tests, including evaluation for gaze and spontaneous nystagmus, (2) positional and positioning tests, and (3) caloric tests.

The ENG examination typically begins with calibrating the patient's eye movement by having the patient perform simple tracking exercises. Typically a light bar is placed between 1 and 2 m in front of the seated patient (Jacobson, Newman, & Kartush, 1993). The patient is asked to track lights as they jump to various positions on the light bar. Calibration targets are usually moved in a predictable fashion, unlike true saccadic testing. The goal of calibration is to be able to assign a value (in degrees) to eccentric eye movements from center (Fig. 5–1).

Current computerized ENG programs have preset distances for both aspects of calibration: distance of the patient from the light bar and distance of the target lights from center. By following this protocol, the computer program can determine whether the patient's eye position differs significantly from the target position. If reasonably accurate calibration cannot be obtained, the test may be performed with a default sensitivity (Norman & Brown, 1999). If default calibration is used, information about vestibular and even oculomotor asymmetry may be gained. Measurements of eye speed and gain would be compromised and could not be applied to normative values.

Evaluation of gaze and spontaneous nystagmus is enhanced through ENG in that visual fixation can be removed, and nystagmus can be recorded and analyzed for intensity and direction. The presence of spontaneous or gaze-evoked nystagmus must be determined before positional or caloric tests as they (1) can affect the recorded intensity of the caloric response, (2) can be mistaken for positional nystagmus, and (3) if strong enough, can skew the results of oculomotor tests. (Interpretation of gaze and spontaneous nystagmus is discussed in Chapter 3.)

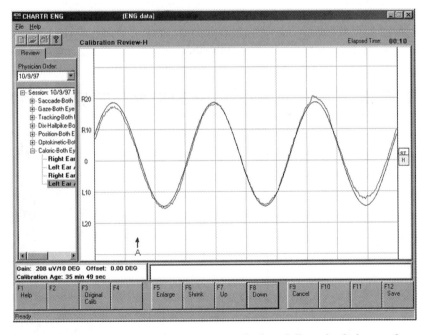

Figure 5–1. Calibration tracing: The patient is asked to follow the lights as they move predictably 10 degrees from center, left and right.

Oculomotor Tests

Oculomotor tests include saccadic tracking, smooth pursuit tracking, and optokinetic tracking. The common bond of these tests is that each one evaluates eye movements that originate in the cerebellum, and abnormalities in these tests are considered signs of neurologic disease. Although certain patterns of abnormality found on oculomotor tests can be suggestive of specific cerebellar lesions, the examiner is cautioned to avoid overinterpreting these results. There are a number of possibilities other than cerebellar dysfunction for poor oculomotor performance. The patient's mental state, fatigue, and a variety of medications can affect oculomotor performance (Cass & Furman, 1993). Oculomotor tests performed with computerized ENG analysis software allow sensitive and documented evaluation. The results of oculomotor tests, when considered with the patient's history and age, can help the health care provider (HCP) in deciding whether neurologic examination or neuroimaging is needed.

Saccades

Saccades are rapid eye movements made to bring an object of interest into the center of the line of sight (foveal vision). Saccadic eye movements are used both voluntarily and reflexively to initiate eye movement quickly toward an object of interest and to stop and "lock on" to the target accurately. Saccades allow patients to refixate their gaze with minimal duration of *retinal slip*. Saccades are tested for (Fig. 5–2) accuracy, *velocity* (eye speed during movement), and *latency* (the difference in time between the presentation of a new target and the initiation of eye movement). Age-weighted normative values for each of these components of saccadic eye movement have been established.

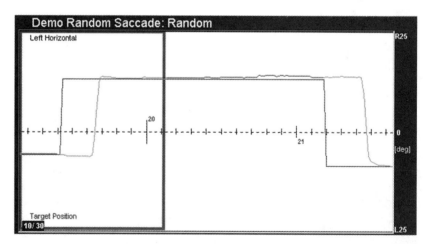

Figure 5–2. Normal saccadic eye movement. This tracing demonstrates a saccade eye movement that is normal in terms of accuracy, velocity, and latency. The eye moves quickly and efficiently to the new target.

The speed of initiation (latency) of a saccade is 150 to 250 ms when the target is unpredictable (random) and about 76 ms with a predictable target (Leigh & Zee, 1991). Latency of saccades is considered abnormal when there is a consistent delay of about 260 to 270 ms or longer. Accuracy of saccades can be affected both before and after the new target has been obtained. Keeping in mind that the goal of a saccadic eye movement is to fixate visually both quickly and accurately on a new object, eye movement that is equal in amplitude to the distance between the former object of interest and the new target is desired. Normal individuals will often "undershoot" the target by about 10 to 15%, referred to as *hypometria* (Fig. 5–3A) and is considered abnormal if saccades are consistently performed at less than about 70% of the target amplitude. Patients with normal cerebellar function will also occasionally overshoot the target. Hypermetria (Fig. 5–3B) is considered abnormal if saccades are consistently more than 15 to 20% over target amplitude. Even when a saccadic eye movement equals the amplitude of the target, for it to

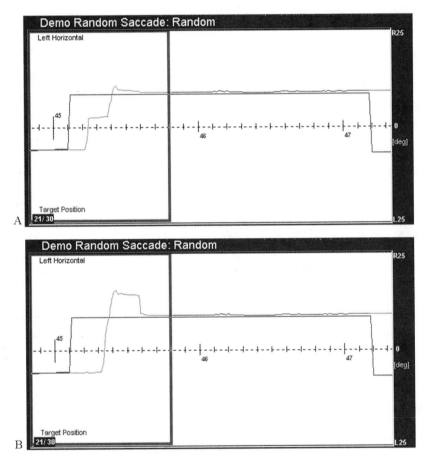

Figure 5–3. Abnormal saccades. (A) Hypometria: the eye stops short of the target and then must make a second corrective saccade to reach the target. (B) Hypermetria: The eye goes past the target, then makes a corrective second saccade back to the target.

be considered normal the eye must be able to remain fixated on the new target. If the eye drifts from or toward (as sometimes occurs in hypometria) the target, it is referred to as a *glissade*.

Saccadic velocity is measured as the peak speed of eye movement when refixating gaze from one target to another (Jacobson et al., 1993). Saccadic velocity is involuntary and has no abnormal upper limit. Peak velocities of saccades have been measured as high as 700 degrees per second and are considered abnormal if consistently slower than 430 degrees per second for large-amplitude saccades (30 degrees) and slower than about 200 degrees per second for small-amplitude saccades (10 degrees) (personal communication, ICS Medical Staff).

The saccade test is performed much like the calibration procedure, with the patient seated and facing a light bar. Unlike the calibration procedure, true saccadic testing must involve a randomly moving target. The patient is instructed to "follow the lights" as accurately as possible while keeping the head still. The lights are moved in a random fashion as controlled by the ENG software. Targets appear on the light bar for 1 to 4 seconds before changing position. The targets may appear anywhere within a range of 30 degrees from center.

Smooth Pursuit

Smooth pursuit eye movements are used to maintain stable gaze on objects that are moving within the visual field. Focus is placed on the object of interest while the background is "blurred." Accurate smooth pursuit requires a target (real or imagined) and matches the velocity (speed) of the target. Smooth-pursuit tracking can function alone or in conjunction with the VOR to assist in gaze stability during movement.

The smooth-pursuit test (also known as *sinusoidal tracking*) is also performed with the patient seated in front of a light bar. Smooth pursuit is evaluated for *symmetry* (the difference between rightward and leftward scores) and *gain* (eye velocity versus target velocity) (Fig. 5–4). Catch-up saccades (rapid eye movements to "catch up" with the target) are effectively eliminated from analysis. Analysis criteria take into consideration significant age and gender effects. Asymmetrical pursuit abilities are highly suggestive of central nervous system (CNS) disease.

A classic example of how the saccadic and pursuit systems work in real life is explained by the following: A flying duck "quacks" and gets your attention, and your saccadic tracking system enables you to look quickly toward and lock on to the duck. Your smooth-pursuit system allows you to follow the duck as it flies across your field of vision.

Optokinetic Tracking

Optokinetic tracking is similar to smooth pursuit tracking in its mechanism of origin. In real life, the optokinetic system starts when the vestibular system fails to "keep up" during sustained head rotation or when the subject is stimulated by full field visual movement with no VOR stimulation. The fluid dynamics of the vestibular apparatus are such that it cannot maintain stimulation of the cupula

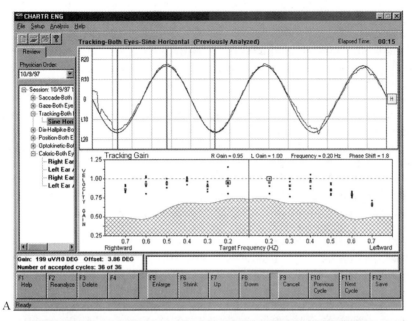

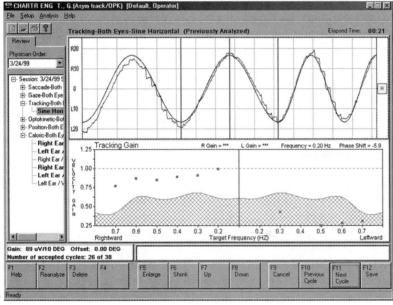

Figure 5–4. Smooth pursuit: (A) The top half of the figure shows the patient's eye movement compared with actual target velocity. The bottom half of the figure shows the analysis pod by ICS Medical. The dots represent the gain of eye movements at various frequencies of target movement (0.2 to 0.7 Hz). The gray area is the abnormal (reduced gain) area. (B) The top half of the figure shows that the patient is unable to follow the target and makes frequent "catch-up" saccades. The bottom half of the figure shows that the gain is abnormal.

during sustained rotation. As the vestibular response gradually decays, the optokinetic and pursuit systems provide input to stabilize the eyes and maintain stable vision.

To maintain visual contact with the environment, eyes make rapid, involuntary corrective saccades toward the oncoming visual scene. After about 30 to 45 seconds, when the vestibular response is exhausted, the optokinetic and pursuit systems are wholly responsible for visual stabilization (Leigh & Zee, 1991). Optokinetic nystagmus can be simulated by exposing the patient to repetitive full-field moving visual stimuli. Various techniques can accomplish this. Older ENG systems frequently supplied an "optokinetic drum," a striped drum that could be spun around in front of the patient. Some laboratories built customized striped drums that would be lowered over the patient's head and spun around to create the repetitive stimuli. Current ENG systems provide optokinetic stimuli by having lights move along the light bar, asking the patient to "count each light" as it passes by. Enclosed rotary-chair systems use a projector to provide full-field (floor to ceiling) stimulation of moving lighted stripes. These are very different tests because patients can easily look away from the light bar, but in full-field stimulation they cannot avoid the moving visual stimulus unless they close their eyes. It has also been demonstrated that the gain (eye velocity) is greater if the patient actively follows the moving targets as opposed to looking passively in the direction of the stimulus (Leigh & Zee, 1991). Kveton, Limb, and Bell (1999) report that standard light-bar stimulation results in a high number of false-positives and question the clinical value of this test as part of the standard ENG battery. Optokinetic tracking is also analyzed (Fig. 5–5) for symmetry and gain.

Positional Tests

Positional tests are performed to determine whether the vestibular system responds normally and symmetrically to changes in head position. Following a peripheral vestibular injury, physiologic adaptation and compensation naturally take place as the brain and brain stem adjust to different resting inputs from the two vestibular end organs. It is understandable that compensation occurs more quickly in the upright resting position because this is the most frequent position of the head. When placed in any different position, dizziness and nystagmus may occur as a result of incomplete compensation in that particular position. In other words, the brain has not acclimated to the unequal inputs generated at that particular position. It is therefore important to detect and measure any spontaneous nystagmus prior to performing positional testing. Position change can exacerbate spontaneous nystagmus. Spontaneous nystagmus that is increased with position change should also diminish with visual fixation.

In performing positional tests, both objective (nystagmus) and subjective (dizziness) responses should be noted. If the patient complains of dizziness and no nystagmus is noted, nonvestibular causes must be considered. Positional nystagmus that beats in the vertical direction, changes directions without position change, or is not suppressed by visual fixation suggests possible brain stem or cerebellar pathology. Smouha and Roussos (1995) report that one fourth of patients with atypical positional nystagmus were found to have CNS disorders

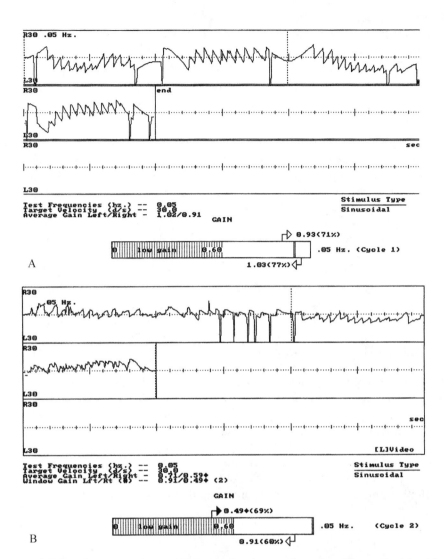

Figure 5–5. Optokinetic tracking: (A) Example of normal tracing. The patient is able to follow smoothly the moving light and then make a quick return saccade to "catch" the next light. (B) Example of abnormal tracing: This patient cannot follow the moving light and makes inefficient saccades to "catch" the next light.

or vascular insufficiency; however, most cases of atypical positional nystagmus are idiopathic and benign. The great majority of positional nystagmus cases are the result of the effects of gravity when head position is changed. Rarely, the nystagmus will be the result of flexion or twisting of the neck (Zee & Fletcher, 1996). The effects of neck flexion must also be ruled out when nystagmus is noted after a position change. The patient should be seated upright. The body can then be pitched forward to simulate the same relative position of head to body while at the same time making sure the head position does not change relative to gravity. If this maneuver elicits nystagmus, then neck flexion must be considered as the cause for the nystagmus as opposed to position change. It should be noted that low-intensity positional nystagmus is noted in many nonsymptomatic patients (McCauley, Dickman, Mustain, & Anand, 1996).

Positioning Tests

Positioning tests are used primarily to determine the presence of BPPV. It is the actual movement into the position that generates the abnormal response rather than the final resting position. The most common form of BPPV results from otolith debris in the posterior semicircular canal. Nystagmus consistent with posterior canal BPPV is torsional (rotary) and is not easily or reliably recorded through electro-oculography (EOG). Because these electrodes record eye movements in the vertical and horizontal planes, torsional eye movement may be missed using this technique. The eyes must be visually observed for nystagmus. Optimally, infrared video goggles (Fig. 5–6) with recording should be used so that eye movements can be documented and reviewed for latency, direction, and duration; however, nystagmus can be easily viewed simply by holding the patient's eyes open and observing. Positioning tests are known as Hallpike, Dix-Hallpike, Barany, or Nylen maneuvers and are performed by having the patient lie quickly into the supine position with the head extended either to the left or the right. The patient should be kept in the test position for 60 seconds and then should sit up quickly. Eye movements should also be monitored upon rising (Epley, 1995). A description of a classic positive response is described in detail in Chapter 6.

Some patients describing a history consistent with BPPV will have negative test results at examination as a result of dispersion of the otoconia *within* the posterior canal. We (the author's clinic) describe this as "probable fatigued BPPV." Lynn and Brey (1993) describe these patients as possibly being in a period of "spontaneous remission" and recommend that the clinician inquire as to when

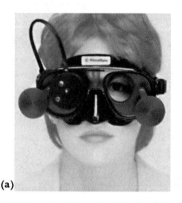
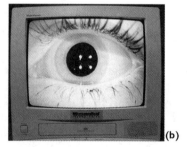

(a)   (b)

Figure 5–6. Infrared video: During positional testing the eye can be monitored for rotary nystagmus that may not be recordable through electro-oculography. (Photo courtesy of Micromedical Technologies.)

the patient last experienced an episode of positional vertigo. If the last episode occurred within the few hours preceding examination, it is suspected that the patient has "probable fatigued BPPV," and we either have the patient reschedule or, depending on travel distance, sit still for an hour or two, after which we will again attempt to provoke an episode of BPPV. Patients who report not having had an episode for several days are suspected of being in a period of "spontaneous remission," and we ask them to contact the clinic if and when the positional vertigo is active. In our clinic, I have found that 49% (48 of 98) of patients suspected by history of having BPPV will have a negative Dix-Hallpike response on the day of initial examination. Of those willing to return for repeat testing (*n* = 25), 44% (14 of 25) had positive Hallpike responses on follow-up testing. Ideally, having patients return to the clinic after they have been careful to avoid any provoking movements for several hours before the examination will increase the chances of provoking an episode in the office. Norre (1994) notes that "a re-examination two to three days later showed a positive vertigo and nystagmus reaction in some cases with positional complaints and negative findings on the first day."

Caloric Testing

Caloric testing is the only test that evaluates the function of one vestibular apparatus at a time. This is done most frequently by irrigating the canal of the test ear with a stream of water. Other stimulation techniques are used. Air and closed-loop (balloon) irrigations may be used (see Chapter 4). The most widely used caloric test technique is that described by Fitzgerald and Hallpike (1942). The patient is placed in the supine 30-degree-angle position so that the horizontal semicircular canal is placed more in the vertical plane for maximum stimulation (Fig. 5–7). The ears are then irrigated with a stream of water that is either 7°C above or 7°C below body temperature. These are done one ear at a time, with a short rest period between irrigations. Caloric stimulation causes a nonphysiologic response in that temperature changes in one ear, which changes the density of endolymph, causes fluid motion and subsequent subjective and physiologic response similar to that which would occur with a slow horizontal head movement.

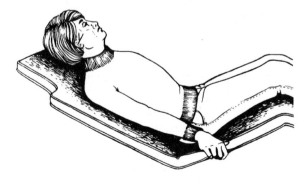

Figure 5–7. A 30-degree supine position: The patient is placed in this supine position during caloric testing. This position vertically orients the horizontal semicircular canal to provide maximal stimulation. (Reprinted with permission from Rubin, W., & Brookler, K. (1991). *Dizziness: etiologic approach to management* (pp. 28–56). New York: Thieme.)

When the patient is placed in the 30-degree supine position, the horizontal semicircular canal lies perpendicular in relation to gravity. The decrease in density of warmer endolymph results in increased endolymph volume. The increased volume causes the endolymph to flow upward through the horizontal canal, toward the cupula. The fluid flow deflects the cupula upward toward the utricle (Baloh & Honrubia, 1990). Because this response is in only one ear, a significant conflict occurs as the nontest ear registers no movement. The resultant response is nystagmus, vertigo, and occasionally nausea, which last for 1 to 2 minutes until the temperature and density of the endolymph return to normal. Most, but not all, patients tolerate caloric testing well. The temperature of the stimulus (warm or cool) determines the direction of fluid flow and subsequent direction of induced nystagmus. Irrigation with warm water (above body temperature) results in an excitatory response on the irrigated side. This results in a slow phase of nystagmus away from the irrigated ear and a fast phase toward the irrigated ear (i.e., warm irrigation on the right results in right beating nystagmus) (Fig. 5–8). Conversely, cool-water irrigation (below body temperature) results in an inhibitory response and fast phase of nystagmus beating away for the irrigated ear. This results in the pneumonic COWS (cold opposite, warm same) as a convenient method of remembering expected caloric results.

The purpose of caloric irrigation is to determine the presence and symmetry of vestibular responsiveness. When no response is obtained to the standard temperature irrigations, ice-water stimulation provides a stronger stimulus and helps to determine whether any residual labyrinthine response exists. Ice-water irrigation does not allow for measures of asymmetry. There are no standards for ice-water irrigation, but 30 to 40 mL over a 20- to 30-second period is typical. Because irrigation lower than body temperature results in an inhibitory response in the supine position, placing the patient in the prone position may result in a stronger excitatory stimulus. My practice is to perform prone irrigations if no response is obtained to supine ice-water irrigation.

It is important to note that standard caloric irrigation temperatures simulate head movement analogous to a speed of approximately 0.002 to 0.004 Hz (cycles of rotation per second) (Baloh, Fife, Furman, & Zee, 1996). The vestibular system

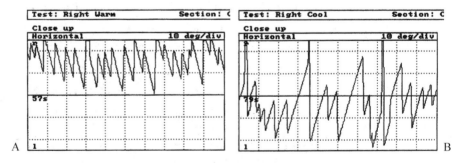

Figure 5–8. Caloric-induced nystagmus: (A) Warm-water irrigation to the right ear results in a right beating nystagmus. (B) Cool water to the right results in a left beating nystagmus.

commonly responds to real-life head movements in the 1- to 6-Hz range (Leigh & Zee, 1991; O'Leary, 1992). A significant vestibular asymmetry can exist in the presence of normal and symmetric caloric responses.

A simple but crude method of determining whether any higher-frequency vestibular function exists in patients with absent caloric response is to roll the patient's head back and forth while observing for nystagmus using EOG, infrared video, or Frenzel lenses. If nystagmus with a fast phase in the same direction of head movement occurs, there is likely some higher frequency vestibular function present, although this technique cannot help in determining whether that response is normal. If no nystagmus occurs while the head is moving, a profound vestibular loss may exist.

Finally, visual fixation should reduce the strength of the caloric response in a patient with intact CNS function. This is evaluated during the period of nystagmus response to caloric stimulation by having the patient stare straight ahead at a light. Whereas there is no established standard for how much caloric-induced nystagmus should suppress with visual fixation, most studies indicate a reduction of 50 to 70% is expected in patients with normal cerebellar function (Alpert, 1974; Jacobson et al., 1993). Failure of fixation suppression can also be tested during rotational testing and will be discussed later in this chapter.

Rotational Test Protocols

Rotational Test Protocols

Rotational chair testing is performed with the patient seated securely in the rotary chair. The head is restrained (Fig. 5–9) to ensure that head movement equals chair movement. The patient wears a seatbelt and harness as well as straps around the ankles to prevent falling out of the chair if the patient becomes dizzy and to avoid any injury. Software programs and test protocols may vary depending on the rotary chair manufacturer and the system purchased. A typical rotary chair protocol includes examination for spontaneous and gaze nystagmus, sinusoidal harmonic acceleration tests at several frequencies, visual–vestibular interaction tests, VOR suppression tests, and step velocity tests.

Evaluation for gaze and spontaneous nystagmus is done before any rotational tests are done because these can create a bias (or asymmetry) in response to the rotary stimulus. The technique for recording these is the same as described earlier for ENG.

Sinusoidal Harmonic Acceleration

Sinusoidal harmonic acceleration (SHA) tests are performed by rotating the patient at specific frequencies, typically ranging from a low of 0.01 Hz to a high of 0.64 Hz. Some rotational chairs can achieve frequencies as high as 1.28 Hz (Shepard, 2001). The rotation stimulus is achieved by a powerful DC servomotor, which is controlled by a computer. The chair can be moved in either direction at a variety of speeds. The frequencies tested are considered "harmonics" or multiples of each other. Each frequency tested is precisely double the speed of the

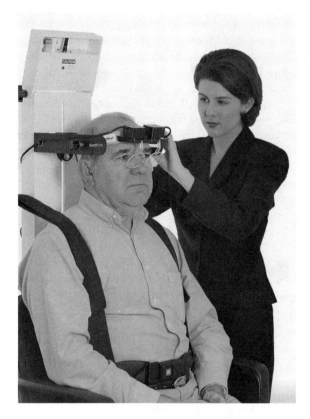

Figure 5–9. Head restraint: The patient's head is securely fastened to the rotational chair to ensure that head movement equals chair movement. (Photo courtesy of Micromedical Technologies.)

previous test frequency. Each frequency is analyzed for gain, phase, and symmetry (Fig. 5–10). It is important to remember that VOR gain for the lower frequencies does not equal head movement. Presumably, because the visual pursuit system augments the VOR response in the lower frequencies, the VOR does not exactly offset head movement. As the speed of head movement increases, gain comes closer to approaching unity gain where eye movement

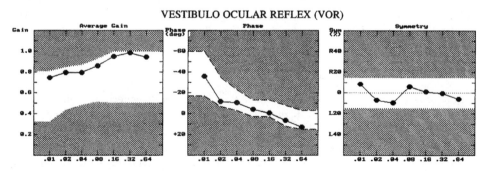

Figure 5–10. Normal sinusoidal harmonic acceleration (SHA) results: Gain, phase and symmetry measures are plotted left to right by increasing frequency.

exactly equals head movement. The results of SHA tests are plotted by frequency and then compared with manufacturer or clinic norms. Results are considered abnormal if two consecutive frequencies fall out of the range of normal.

Patients with acute unilateral vestibular dysfunction often display spontaneous nystagmus in darkness which can create a bias and lead to an asymmetry, often but not always, toward the side of the suspected lesion. Gain will also be reduced. As vestibular compensation occurs, both symmetry and gain tend to return toward normal within several days. Phase may remain abnormal even after compensation occurs, and abnormal phase is the most common positive finding in SHA testing. Patients with bilateral vestibular loss will usually demonstrate decreased gain at affected frequencies (Fig. 5–11). Occasionally, the VOR gain will actually exceed the velocity of head movement. This suggests the possibility of cerebellar dysfunction (Furman & Cass, 1996). Therapy exercises designed to improve the VOR (described in Chapter 6) would be appropriate for attempting to reduce asymmetry and increase gain of the VOR.

Visual–Vestibular Interaction Tests

Visual–vestibular interaction tests (VVORs) are performed by having the patient view objects or stripes on the wall as the rotational chair moves in a clockwise and then in a counterclockwise direction. In this situation the patient uses a combination of VOR and visual pursuit to track efficiently the objects or stripes. The goal is to effectively match eye speed to the speed of rotation, and so a normal score should approach unity gain (a gain of 1). In patients with deficient VOR at the same frequency tested for VVOR, a normal score demonstrates that the patient is able to compensate for the deficient VOR with voluntary pursuit. Decreased gain on the VVOR test is suggestive of dysfunction in the cerebellum or brain stem (Furman & Cass, 1996). Although improvement in smooth-pursuit tracking has not been demonstrated as a benefit of vestibular therapy, a variety of vestibular exercises may promote compensatory eye tracking strategies.

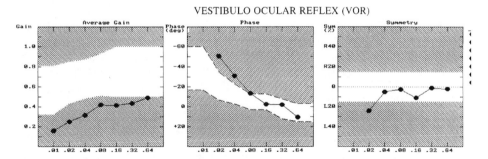

Figure 5–11. Abnormal sinusoidal harmonic acceleration (SHA) results. This patient, diagnosed with bilateral vestibular hypofunction secondary to the use of gentamicin, demonstrates reduced gain across all frequencies. When gain measurements are very low (as above), phase measurements must be interpreted with caution.

Vestibular Ocular Reflex Suppression Test

Vestibular ocular reflex suppression test (VFX) examines the patient's ability to suppress vestibular-induced eye movements through visual fixation. The patient is asked to fixate visually on a target that rotates at the same speed as the chair. The target stimulus can be achieved through a laser target rotating with the chair, or the patient can simply hold the thumb out and stare at it during the rotations. This is essentially the same test that is performed during caloric stimulation and should be normal in patients with intact cerebellar function. A normal score would result in at least 90% suppression of the VOR gain.

Improvement in suppression of the VOR through visual fixation as a result of vestibular therapy has not been demonstrated. Vestibular therapy is therefore not appropriate when abnormal VFX testing is the only noted abnormality. Appropriate follow-up would involve ruling out significant neurologic disease through neuroimaging or neurologic consultation.

Step Velocity Tests

Step velocity tests involve impulsive acceleration that is sustained in one direction for approximately 45 seconds. The chair is then abruptly stopped. A nystagmus response is produced by the acceleration, and the slow component velocity is recorded. The intensity of the nystagmus response (described as per rotary nystagmus) will gradually decrease over the period of sustained rotation. The point (in seconds) at which the slow component velocity decreases to 37% of its peak is labeled the *time constant*. This measure not only records the physiologic response of the horizontal semicircular canal but also measures the velocity storage mechanism. The velocity storage mechanism describes a continuation of neural response which persists after the fluid dynamics of the labyrinth have been exhausted (velocity storage is discussed in Chapter 3 under Headshake Nystagmus). A normal time constant is within 12 to 14 seconds (Fig. 5–12). Typically, the nystagmus response will continue to decrease after this period and will cease completely before the end of a 45-second sustained

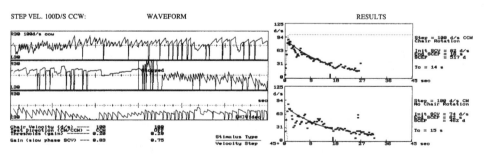

Figure 5–12. Normal step velocity test: The trace shows the nystagmus response to counterclockwise chair movement. When the chair suddenly stops rotating after 45 seconds, a nystagmus response in the opposite direction occurs. Step velocity tests measure the time taken for the slow phase velocity of this nystagmus response to diminish.

rotation. When the chair abruptly stops, a nystagmus response (postrotary nystagmus) in the opposite direction will occur. A time constant is also measured for this response. Gain (slow phase of nystagmus velocity divided by chair velocity) is also measured. Normal results typically fall within 0.4 to 0.7 gain units.[2] Decreased time constant and reduced gain on step velocity testing are sensitive but nonlocalizing findings for vestibular dysfunction (Furman & Cass, 1996). Vestibular therapy may increase the gain on step velocity tests, but reduced time constant (like phase) is often a lasting abnormal legacy of vestibular injury.

Active Head Rotation

The active head rotation test (AHR) is described in Chapter 4. The patient, once seated and fit with the appropriate hardware, is asked to rotate the head back and forth in the yaw plane while staring at a target 1 to 2 m in front. This stimulates the horizontal semicircular canals. Unlike any other vestibular function tests, AHR can provide information about the function of the vertical VOR as well, completed by having patients shake their head up and down in the pitch plane. This motion stimulates both the posterior and anterior semicircular canals. The speed of head rotation is determined by patients attempting to move their head in time to a computer-generated tone that increases in frequency over a 15- to 18-second period. The manufacturers of AHR equipment recommend that at least three sweeps or tests be performed in each direction of head movement to eliminate artifact and give a better average of VOR response. Because the AHR test involves short, rapid head movements, only the slow phase of nystagmus is produced. These are then measured for gain, phase, and symmetry (Fig. 5–13). AHR should not be performed in patients with a history of severe neck injury. As in rotational chair testing, decreases in gain and any noted asymmetry may be improved by vestibular therapy designed to enhance the VOR. Abnormal phase values do not typically improve as a result of therapy.

Posturography

The term *posturography* may be used to describe any test of postural stability or standing balance; however, the term is most often used to describe computerized dynamic posturography (CDP) by Neurocom. Several different posturography techniques are described in Chapter 4. Several studies have attempted to estimate the specificity and sensitivity of the Equitest (DiFabio, 1995; Evans & Krebs, 1999). These studies have mostly proved frustrating or confusing because posturography cannot be compared with tests of vestibular function and because no "gold standard" exists by which to determine the accuracy of the results. Furman (1995) points out that posturography attempts to evaluate the vestibulospinal reflex, whereas rotational chair and ENG specifically evaluate the

---

[2]Gain units represent a ratio of eye velocity compared to chair or head velocity. If the velocity of the eye equals the velocity of the chair or head, then the gain is 1 (a 1:1 ratio). If the eye movement velocity equals only 80% of the head or chair velocity, the gain would be 0.8 (a 0.8:1 ratio).

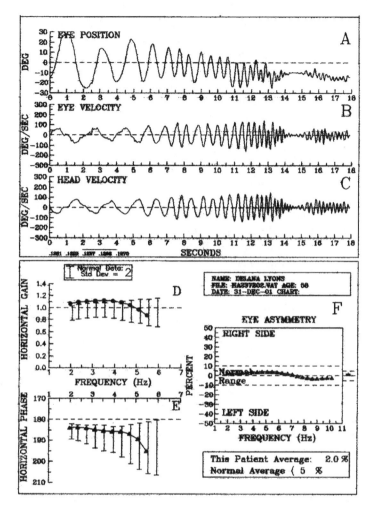

Figure 5–13. Active head rotation recording: The top half of the figure shows (in descending order) average eye position, eye velocity raw data, and head velocity raw data over an 18-second sweep. The lower half of the figure shows the patient's response compared with norms obtained for gain, phase, and symmetry.

horizontal VOR. He also postulates that vestibular influences on postural sway probably involve the vertical VOR and that posturography augments the evaluation of vestibular patients by evaluating structures overlooked in tests of the VOR.

Postural stability (balance) requires harmonious and synchronous integration of information sent by the peripheral sensors (vestibular, vision, and somatosensory) and received at the cerebellum. Standing balance is primarily dependent on the somatosensory feedback obtained from the stretch receptors in the muscles of lower legs as well as contributions from the ankle, knee, and hip joints. In situations where somatosensory feedback may be impaired or unavailable, such as patients with peripheral neuropathy of the lower extremities or normal patients standing on a compliant surface, vestibular and visual information must be used to supplement proprioceptive information to maintain balance. Following an injury to any of the peripheral sensors, CNS compensation may cause an increased reliance on the remaining intact sensors. For example, a patient with a vestibular injury may become overly reliant on visual feedback for the maintenance of balance. As long as visual feedback is available and reliable, balance is maintained. When this patient is inevitably exposed to a situation where visual feedback is unavailable (in the dark) or unreliable (busy visual environment such as a crowded store), balance and orientation may be compromised.

Computerized dynamic posturography has been developed as a means to evaluate the relative contribution of each of the peripheral sensors as they relate to postural stability. CDP is not a diagnostic site of lesion test but is rather an assessment of functional balance under a variety of conditions. The two subtests performed in CDP are the sensory organization test (SOT) and the motor control test (MCT). The SOT, which is described in detail in Chapter 4, involves measurement of postural stability or sway while systematically removing or distorting visual and somatosensory information used for balance. The six conditions are described in Table 5–1.

Various patterns of performance have been associated with specific functional impairments (Fig. 5–14). A vestibular dysfunction pattern is referred to as a "5, 6" pattern. This means that the patient was unable to maintain postural control in conditions 5 and 6 of the SOT where both visual and somatosensory cues are absent or distorted. In this situation, the patient must rely on vestibular information for maintenance of balance. If vestibular signals are compromised, the patient has insufficient information to maintain postural stability. As the vestibular patient undergoes central compensation, the likelihood of displaying a "5, 6" pattern decreases (Fetter, Deiner, & Dichgans, 1991). Patients exhibiting

Table 5–1. Six Conditions of Sensory Organization Testing

Condition One— Stable platform with eyes open in a stable visual environment (patient has full use of all information: visual, vestibular, and somatosensory)

Condition Two— Stable platform with eye closed (patient must rely on vestibular and somatosensory information)

Condition Three— Stable platform with moving visual surround (patient must suppress a false sense of visually induced movement and rely on vestibular and somatosensory inputs)

Condition Four— Unstable platform with eyes open in a stable visual environment (patient must rely on vestibular and visual inputs)

Condition Five— Unstable platform with eyes closed (patient must rely on vestibular input only because visual and somatosensory feedback have been eliminated)

Condition Six— Unstable platform and unstable visual environment (patient must rely on vestibular input alone and suppress a false sense of visually induced movement)

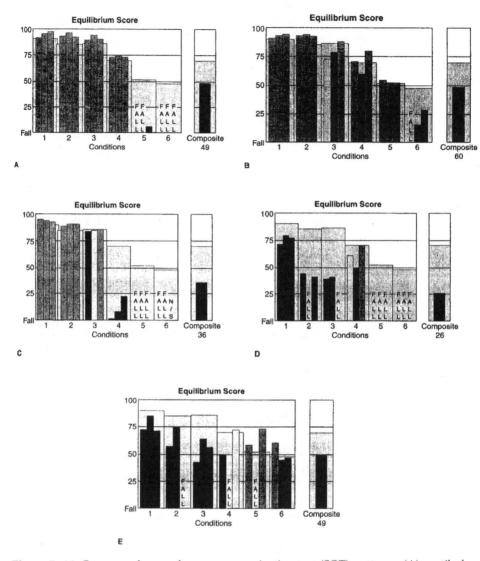

Figure 5–14. Common abnormal sensory organization test (SOT) patterns. (A) vestibular dysfunction; (B) vision preference; (C) somatosensory dependent; (D) vision dependent; (E) aphysiologic.

this pattern are candidates for vestibular therapy designed to stimulate the VOR and reduce dependency on visual information.

A "visual preference" (3, 6) pattern indicates that the patient makes use of all three senses (vision, vestibular, and somatosensory) but relies on false visual information and loses balance in the sway reference conditions (SOT conditions 3 and 6). When vision is removed, the patient is able to deal effectively with the same decreased somatosensory feedback (condition 5). This pattern does not suggest vestibular dysfunction. Nashner (1993) suggests that this pattern may be suggestive of abnormal central processing of vestibular and visual information. These patients are not good candidates for vestibular therapy, and referral for neurologic evaluation is indicated.

A "surface dependence" or "somatosensory dependence" pattern has been suggested when the patient is unable to maintain postural stability when somatosensory feedback is distorted (conditions 4, 5, and 6). These patients have difficulty when somatosensory information is decreased under all the previously described visual conditions. These patients should be referred for physical therapy or neurologic assessment of strength and sensation in the lower extremities.

A "visual dependence" pattern suggests that the patient may be overly reliant on visual information for maintenance of balance. These patients are able to maintain postural stability with both reliable and distorted somatosensory feedback as long as stable visual information is available (conditions 1 and 4). When visual information is either removed or distorted, the subjects lose postural stability (conditions 2, 3, 5, and 6). Therapy that incorporates a gradual reduction in visual feedback while performing exercises may reduce visual dependency for balance.

An "aphysiologic" pattern has been described (also described as a nonspecific pattern) when the patient demonstrates better postural ability on the more difficult conditions. Theoretically, a patient feigning a balance disorder has better control and can feign increased sway in the simpler conditions. In the later conditions (5 and 6) even normal patients may have to exert some effort to maintain stability. Minimally, this pattern would be difficult to explain clinically. Additionally, "aphysiologic" patients tend to show greater inter-test variability compared with normal or vestibular patients performing to the best of their ability (Cevette, Puetz, Marion, Wertz, & Muenter, 1995). In cases of suspected malingering, this pattern provides some objective evidence to support clinical suspicion. Nashner (1993) provides an in-depth discussion of the theoretical implications of various patterns on SOT.

The MCT involves recording the patient's response to small, brief movements of the support surface. Measurements of response latency and symmetry are compared with established norms. Patients with vestibular dysfunction typically have responses within the normal range. Abnormalities in latency or symmetry are suggestive of CNS disorders that affect the long-loop pathways from the lower extremities (DiFabio, 1995).

Allum and Shepard (1999) suggest five different types of patients that may benefit from posturography:

1. Patients exhibiting or complaining of chronic dysequilibrium and postural instability but with normal clinical examinations
2. Patients whom the examiner suspects may be malingering
3. Patients with possible cervicogenic dysequilibrium (i.e., head trauma, whiplash injuries, and such)
4. Patients suspected of multifactorial dysequilibrium secondary to age-related decreased efficiency of the CNS and peripheral sensory systems responsible for balance
5. Patients with apparent poorly compensated vestibular injuries

Hussam, Shepard, Asher, Smith-Wheelock, and Telian (1998) compared several clinical measures of equilibrium and found that both Equitest and the clinical test for sensory integration and balance (CTSIB) (described in Chapter 4) proved useful in identifying patients with abnormal postural control. Many clinics cannot afford or justify the expense of the Equitest, but some form of posturography can be completed at minimal expense.

References

Allum, H. J., & Shepard, N. T. (1999). An overview of the clinical use of dynamic posturography in the differential diagnosis of balance disorders. *J Vestib Res*, 9, 223–252.

Alpert, J. (1974). Failure of fixation suppression: a pathologic effect of vision on caloric nystagmus. *Neurology*, 24, 891–896.

Andrews, J., & Honrubia, V. (1996). Meniere's disease. In: R. Baloh, & G. M. Halmagyi, (Eds.), *Disorders of the vestibular system* (pp. 300–317). New York: Oxford University Press.

Baloh, R.W., Fife, T., Furman, J., & Zee, D. (1996). *Neurotology. Continuum: lifelong learning in neurology*, 2(2).

Baloh, R. W., & Honrubia, V. (1990). *Clinical neurophysiology of the vestibular system*, 2nd ed. Philadelphia: F.A. Davis.

Cass, S., & Furman, J. (1993). Medications and their effects on vestibular testing. ENG Report. *ICS Medical*, 81–84.

Cevette, M. J., Puetz, B., Marion, M. S., Wertz, M. L., & Muenter, M. D. (1995). Aphysiologic performance on dynamic posturography. *Otolaryngol Head Neck Surg*, 112(6), 676–688.

DiFabio, R. P. (1995). Sensitivity and specificity of platform posturography for identifying patients with vestibular dysfunction. *Phys Ther*, 75(4), 290–305.

Epley, J. (1995). Positional vertigo related to canalithiasis. *Otolaryngol Head Neck Surg*, 112(1), 154–161.

Evans, M. K., & Krebs, D. E. (1999). Posturography does not test vestibulospinal function. *Otolaryngol Head Neck Surg*, 120, 164–173.

Ferraro, J. (2000). Electrocochleography. In: Roeser, R. J., Valente, M., & Hosford–Dunn, H. (Eds.), *Audiology: diagnosis* (pp. 425–450). New York: Thieme.

Fetter, M., Deiner, H. C., & Dichgans, J. (1991). Recovery of postural control after an acute unilateral vestibular lesion in humans. *J Vestib Res*, 1, 373–383.

Fitzgerald, G., & Hallpike, C. S. (1942). Studies in human vestibular function: Observations on the directional preponderance ("nystagmusbereitschaft") of caloric nystagmus resulting from cerebral lesions. *Brain*, 62(2), 115–137.

Flickinger-Moorehead, J., & Downs, M. (1993). Audiology: Its role in the dizzy patient. In: I. K. Arenberg (Ed.), *Dizziness and balance disorders* (pp. 453–459). New York: Kugler Publications.

Furman, J. (1995). Role of posturography in the management of vestibular patients. *Otolaryngol Head Neck Surg*, 112(1), 8–15.

Furman, J., & Cass, S. (1996). Laboratory evaluation: electronystagmography and rotational testing. In: R. W. Baloh, & G. M. Halmagyi (Eds.), *Disorders of the vsestibular system* (pp. 191–210). New York: Oxford University Press.

Hussam, E. K., Shepard, N. T., Asher, A. M., Smith-Wheelock, M., & Telian, S. A. (1998). Evaluation of clinical measures of equilibrium. *Laryngoscope*, 108, 311–319.

Jacobson, G., Newman, C., & Kartush, J. (1993). *Handbook of balance function testing*. St. Louis: Mosby Year Book.

Jerger, J., & Jordan, C. (1980). Normal audiometric findings. *Am J Otol*, 1(3), 157–158.

Keim, R. J. (1985). The pitfalls of limiting ENG testing to patients with vertigo. *Laryngoscope*, 59, 1208–1212.

Kveton, J. F., Limb, C. J., & Bell, M. D. (1999). Comparison of optokinetic nystagmus elicited by full versus partial field stimulation: diagnostic implication. *Otolaryngol Head Neck Surg*, 121(1), 52–56.

Lee, C. S., Paparella, M. M., Margolis, R. H., & Le, C. (1995). Audiological profiles and Meniere's disease. *Ear Nose Throat J*, 74(8), 527–532.

Leigh, R. J., & Zee, D. (1991). *The neurology of eye movements,* 2nd ed. Philadelphia: F.A. Davis.

Lynn, S., & Brey, R. (1993). Benign paroxysmal positional vertigo with indeterminate cerebellar lesion: case report. *J Am Acad Audiol, 4,* 384–391.

McCauley, J., Dickman, D., Mustain, W., & Anand, V. (1996). Positional nystagmus in asymptomatic human subjects. *Otolaryngol Head Neck Surg, 114,* 545–553.

Martin, G. K., Ohlms, L. A., Franklin, D. J., Harris, F. P., & Lonsbury-Martin, B. L. (1990). Distortion-product emissions in humans. In: M. S. Robinette, & T. J. Glattke (Eds.), *Otoacoustic emissions* (pp. 151–180). New York: Thieme.

Nashner, L. (1993). Computerized dynamic posturography: Clinical applications. In: G. Jacobson, C. Newman, & J. Kartush, J. (Eds.), *Handbook of balance function testing* (pp. 308–334). St. Louis: Mosby Year Book.

National Institute of Health (NIH) (1991). Acoustic neuroma. Consensus statement. NIH Consensus Development Conference, Dec 11–13, 1991. Vol. 9, No. 4.

Norman, M., & Brown, E. (1999). Variations in calibration for computerized electronystagmography. *Br J Audiol, 33*(1), 1–7.

Norre, M. E. (1994). Relevance of function tests in the diagnosis of vestibular disorders. *Clin Otolaryngol, 19,* 433–440.

Ohlms, L.A., Lounsbery-Martin, B. L., & Martin, G. K. (1991). Acoustic distortion products: Separation of sensory from neural dysfunction in sensorineural hearing in human beings and rabbits. *Otolaryngol Head Neck Surg, 104,* 159–174.

O'Leary, D. P. (1992). Physiological bases and a technique for testing the full range of vestibular function. *Rev Laryngol, 113*(5), 407–412.

Robinette, M. S., Bauch, C. D., Olsen, W. O., & Cevette, M. J. (2000). Auditory brainstem response and magnetic resonance imaging for acoustic neuromas. *Arch Otolaryngol Head Neck Surg, 126*(8), 963–966.

Rubin, W., & Brookler, K. (1991). *Dizziness: Etiologic approach to management* (pp. 28–56). New York: Thieme Medical Publishers.

Schmidt, R. J., Sataloff, R. T., Newman, J., Spiegel, J. R., & Myers, D. L. (2001). The sensitivity of auditory brainstem response testing for the diagnosis of acoustic neuromas. *Arch Otolaryngol Head Neck Surg, 127,* 19–22.

Shelton, C., Harnsbarger, H. R., Allen, R., & King, B. (1996). Fast spin echo magnetic resonance imaging: Clinical application in screening for acoustic neuroma. *Otolaryngol Head Neck Surg, 114,* 71–76.

Shepard, N. (2001). Rotational chair testing. In: J. Goebel, (Ed.), *Practical management of the dizzy patient* (pp. 129–142). Philadelphia: Lippincott–Williams & Wilkins.

Silman, S. (1984). *The acoustic reflex: Basic principles and clinical applications.* New York: Academic Press.

Smouha, E. E., & Roussos, C. (1995). Atypical forms of paroxysmal positional nystagmus. *Ear Nose Throat J, 74,* 649–656.

Yellin, M. W., Waller, M., & Roland, P. S. (1993). Dehydration testing and the diagnosis of Meniere's disease: case report. *J Am Acad Audiol, 4,* 432–436.

Zee, D. S., & Fletcher, W. A. (1996). Bedside examination. In: R. W. Baloh, & G. M. Halmagyi, (Eds.), *Disorders of the vestibular system* (pp. 178–190). New York: Oxford University Press.

6

Treatment of Vestibular Dysfunction

Historical Perspective

Treatment for vestibular disorders has historically fallen into three categories: (1) medical treatment of symptoms and underlying pathologic conditions; (2) surgical stabilization of the end organ or vestibular nerve through reparative or ablative techniques; and (3) observation, reassurance, and counseling to "learn to live with it."

Vestibular rehabilitation (VR) offers an alternative form of treatment to many patients who previously would have fallen into one of these three categories. Treatment of vestibular disorders through exercise and repositioning techniques has gained popularity within the last decade, and recent literature supports the efficacy of these approaches. The concept of an exercise or rehabilitation approach to dizziness and balance disorders is not new. British otolaryngologist Terrance Cawthorne is the earliest documented proponent of an exercise approach in treating patients with vestibular symptoms. Cawthorne (1945a,b) published articles describing the complexity of the balance system and the relationship between the vestibular system and visual and somatosensory inputs. In his early writings, Cawthorne discussed the benefits of activity and exercise in recovery from "vestibular injuries." He noted that following unilateral labyrinthectomy active patients seemed to recover faster and more completely than did more sedate patients.

Cawthorne, along with physiologist Dr. F. S. Cooksey (1945), developed a series of exercises, currently known as *Cawthorne–Cooksey exercises*, thought to promote central compensation and habituation through repetition of symptom-provoking maneuvers. These exercises established the basic framework of current VR programs. Concepts such as critical periods of compensation following injury, the need to provide the patient with progressively more difficult exercises, and the need to reduce functional disability are all addressed (Cooksey, 1945). Little progress occurred in the acceptance of exercise as a treatment option over the 25 years following Cawthorne (1945a,b) and Cooksey's (1945) original articles.

During the 1970s and early 1980s, a flurry of activity produced several articles that expanded on the theories of the vestibular compensation process and that reintroduced the concept of vestibular exercises (Hood, 1970; Pfaltz, 1983; Pfaltz & Kamath, 1971).

McCabe, in 1970, expanded on Cawthorne's ideas and described "labyrinthine exercises" as "our most useful single tool in the alleviation of protracted recurrent vertigo." He advocated the importance of patient education and the need for proper stimulus to allow the brain to "get over" vestibular loss. McCabe described the two peripheral vestibular apparatuses as "partners," and his explanation regarding vestibular exercises is worth repeating:

1.   Exclude through careful investigation progressive neurologic, otologic, or other disease.
2.   Explain to the patient the nature of his disorder. He has a disease of the balance center and
     a.   The two balance centers are partners, and they work not against but with each other.
     b.   In this disorder, one partner cannot carry his share of the load.
     c.   At certain times a comparison of partners occurs, and one is found wanting – then trouble (vertigo) ensues.
     d.   The longer the two partners ignore each other, the more major the trouble is going to be when they meet.
     e.   The closer and more often the two partners confront each other with the problem they mutually want to solve (dysequilibrium); the more quickly it will be solved.
     f.   When the partners reach an agreement which is mutual, balance results.
3.   Give to the patient on the basis of the above rationale a series of instructions, which he can carry out pertinent to the nature, and severity of his symptoms and his disease. You do not have a life-threatening process. Your symptoms are only as important to the degree to which they annoy you. You will in time master them: when you do, they will be gone.

McCabe goes on to note that medications strong enough to suppress symptoms might also "prevent or delay the reparative process."

Hecker, Haug, and Herndon (1974) reported the results of Cawthorne–Cooksey exercises on a group of patients they considered to be "vestibular types." They, however, included patients believed to have vertigo from vascular insufficiency and those with "Hallpike-type vertigo." They found that 84% of these patients treated with such exercises reported improvement. In this study, the authors believed that the failures were due to the lack of patient compliance or emotional distress.

Norre and DeWeert (1980) also proposed a therapy program for patients with peripheral vestibular disorders based on the concept of habituation. They selected only patients with what they described as "provoked" vertigo, or vertigo elicited only by movement. These patients were instructed to perform repetitive maneuvers that elicited vertigo. More than 50% of the patients in this study were considered to have paroxysmal positional vertigo (described later in this chapter). Ninety-one percent of their cases reported "some improvement," whereas 64% reported more than a 75% reduction in symptoms. A small control group demonstrated lack of improvement from "sham" exercises, but after changing their program to include habituation or provoking movement, improvement was noted. Failure to perform the prescribed exercises correctly was considered a major factor in the finding of little improvement in some patients. They found no significant effect related to delaying initiation of therapy following onset of symptoms.

Margaret Dix (1984) promoted the concept of VR in the United Kingdom with numerous publications during the 1980s. She emphasized encouragement, motivation, and patient education as critical factors for success. She based her therapy program on the original Cawthorne–Cooksey exercises but adds, "The rationale, then, of head exercises in vestibular disorders is to provoke deliberately and systematically as many spells of vertigo as can be tolerated."

A common bond between most of the published reports of this era is the emphasis on intentionally provoking symptoms by creating an error signal or sensory conflict (Pfaltz, 1983). In theory, cerebellar or "adaptive" plasticity works to integrate what is initially perceived as abnormal and through repetition and motor learning (habituation) interprets the vestibular signals as normal. Adaptive plasticity refers to the brain's ability to modify the amount (or gain) of the vestibular ocular reflex to minimize visual–vestibular conflict. Sensory conflicts occur when there is disagreement between incoming (afferent) information regarding movement, balance, and orientation, which can occur when there is an asymmetric response between the two labyrinths in response to head movement or when there is a disagreement (or conflict) between vestibular, visual, or proprioceptive input. An example of sensory conflict would be the frequently described sensation of movement or disorientation that occurs while sitting in a car next to a large truck or bus. The size of the truck or bus allows full visual field stimulation. When the truck or bus moves forward, there is a brief illusory sensation that one is moving backward. Those with a healthy vestibular system quickly prioritize the incoming information and rely on the vestibular response indicating lack of movement. Patients with vestibular weakness may not react quickly or appropriately and lose balance or orientation.

Controversies in Vestibular Rehabilitation

The science of vestibular testing and treatment is still in a relative infancy stage. Many areas of disagreement and controversy exist. At this time, no "gold standard" test has been established to provide a conclusive diagnosis in many vestibular patients. As a result, sensitivity and specificity of various vestibular tests can not be determined. Past studies on the effectiveness of various treatment techniques often combined patients with stable vestibular insufficiency with patients experiencing only provoked vertigo (see section on benign paroxysmal positional vertigo [BPPV]). Despite evidence suggesting that VR is more effective and medication is less effective for most chronically dizzy patients, most dizzy patients are still treated with medication. The following section reviews literature pertaining to some of these areas of controversy.

Critical Periods of Compensation

The existence of critical periods of compensation for vestibular compensation is unresolved. Animal studies have focused on the effects of physical activity and visual stimulation on the rate and extent of recovery following vestibular deafferentation. Lacour, Roll, and Appaix (1976) performed unilateral vestibular neurectomy on a population of baboons. The legs of one group were restrained by a plaster cast for 4 days; a second group was allowed freedom of movement. Rate of recovery measured by locomotor ataxia (difficulty walking) was significantly delayed in the restrained group. Mathog and Peppard (1982) reported a 58 to 70% faster rate of recovery following unilateral labyrinthectomy in cats forced into exercise than cats without exercise. Exercise in this study essentially involved allowing the cat freedom to walk about the laboratory as opposed to being restricted to a cage. Squirrel monkeys forced into activity by means of a motor-driven rotating cage recovered from unilateral labyrinthectomy significantly faster than monkeys left to recover naturally (Igarashi, Levy, O-Uchi, & Reschke, 1981).

Cats kept in the dark following unilateral labyrinthectomy showed a reduced gain of the vestibular ocular reflex (VOR) and a persistence of spontaneous nystagmus (representing a tonic imbalance in the vestibular system) compared with a control group exposed to light. Gain increased and spontaneous nystagmus quickly diminished when the same cats were allowed exposure to light (Courjon, Jeannerod, Ossuzio, & Schmid, 1977). Whereas this effectively demonstrates the role of vision in vestibular adaptation, it does not support the concept of critical periods of compensation. A similar study performed on guinea pigs showed that total visual deprivation following labyrinthectomy had no effect on spontaneous nystagmus (Smith, Darlington, & Curthoys, 1986). This indicates the possibility of species specific patterns of compensation and casts some caution toward using animal studies to predict the mechanisms of vestibular adaptation in humans. Human studies on the subject have been contradictory. Several investigators found that the final outcomes were similar when delaying therapy to a specific group of patients (Norre & DeWeert, 1980; Szturm, Ireland, & Lessing-Turner, 1994).

Rehabilitation versus Repositioning

Brandt and Daroff (1980), based on the principles of habituation, promoted the use of provocative movements for the treatment of BPPV. They reported dramatic benefits from the prescribed exercise but considered the rate of recovery to be too fast to be the result of centrally mediated habituation or central nervous system (CNS) compensation. They speculated that the exercises "provided a mechanical means to promote loosening and ultimate dispersion of the otolithic debris from the cupula." The recommended movements are strikingly similar to those recommended by Semont, Freyss, and Vitte (1988) in their description of their technique for the liberatory maneuver. Norre and Beckers (1987, 1988) compared the relative effectiveness of medications, vestibular habituation therapy (VHT) and what they described as the "brisk method" of treating patients with diagnosed BPPV. The brisk method is similar to the Semont maneuver, and the authors refer to the work of Toupet and Semont (1985) in describing the maneuver. They found VHT to be significantly more effective than vestibular suppressant medication in reducing the complaints and nystagmus response of BPPV. Additionally, the brisk method resulted in a reduction of positional vertigo in 52% of patients, whereas 32% of VHT patients had similar improvement at 1 week after treatment. This study demonstrates that patients with BPPV benefit from single-treatment procedures more quickly than from traditional habituation therapy. Improvement was based on both the patient's subjective sensation of vertigo and the presence of nystagmus typically associated with BPPV. Single-treatment approaches to BPPV are discussed later in this chapter.

In contrast to some earlier research, which included patients with BPPV in studies thought to be measuring adaptation and habituation, most of the more recent research has excluded these patients, limiting subjects to patients believed to suffer from chronic peripheral vestibulopathy (stable and permanent vestibular dysfunction).

Vestibular Rehabilitation versus Medication

Three more recent studies demonstrate the efficacy of exercises versus medication in improving postural control in vestibular deficient patients. Horak, Jones-Rycewicz, Black, and Shumway-Cook (1992) compared "relative effectiveness of VR, general conditioning exercises, and vestibular suppressant medication" on subjective dizziness and postural control. Postural control was measured by sensory organization testing (SOT) (see Chapters 4 and 5) and timed one-leg standing with eyes open and closed. VR consisted of intensive (twice per week) sessions with a physical therapist, performing exercises customized to the patient's specific complaints. General conditioning consisted of similar intensive therapy sessions with strength, range of motion, and cardiac fitness as the therapy goals. These exercises were nonspecific to the patient's complaints. The medication group was treated with Valium or meclizine, both centrally sedating medications. Over a 6-week treatment period, all groups reported a reduction in symptoms, but only the VR group showed significant objective improvement in scores obtained from SOT and standing balance tests.

Fujino et al. (1996) reported differences in subjective improvement in clinical signs and symptoms in two groups. One group was treated with medication only (betahistine, a histamine analog believed to stimulate circulation in the inner ear), with instructions to "take a rest" during the study period. This medication, betahistine, was previously shown to reduce the severity of dizziness in patients with peripheral vestibular-induced vertigo. A second group was treated with the same medication but concurrently treated with a modified version of Cawthorne–Cooksey exercises. Over an 8-week period, Fujino et al. (1996) noted significantly greater improvement in the exercise group.

The use of centrally sedating medication may in fact impede the benefits of VR therapy. Shepard, Telian, and Smith-Wheelock (1990) reported that patients taking vestibular suppressants, antidepressants, tranquilizers, and anticonvulsants ultimately achieve the same level of compensation as patients not taking similar medications, but the length of therapy is significantly longer.

Generic versus Customized Exercise

Cawthorne–Cooksey exercises had been used as the standard treatment for vestibular patients and had been used in most studies designed to demonstrate the efficacy of an exercise approach to treating these patients. More recently, investigators examined the relative benefits of a more customized approach, designing specific exercises for each patient based on complaints and diagnosis.

Szturm et al. (1994) reported the findings of a study comparing two groups. One group was treated with an intensive customized exercise program designed to produce retinal slip and increase postural control. The second group received Cawthorne–Cooksey exercises on a home program basis. Performance was measured both before and after SOT and rotary chair testing. The customized group showed a significant improvement in standing balance performance and in reducing VOR asymmetry. The home-based program group showed no significant improvement in either test. Patients placed originally in the home-based group, eventually provided with the customized exercises, ultimately displayed improvement similar to that of the original custom exercise group. This study demonstrates the efficacy of intensive customized treatment using objective measures and demonstrates the benefit of customized versus generic vestibular exercises.

Shepard and Telian (1995) in a similar study found that 84% of chronic vestibular patients treated with an exercise program customized to the patients' needs reported complete or dramatic improvement, whereas 64% of patients treated with generic exercise reported similar improvement. Objectively, the customized exercise group demonstrated significantly improved performance on a number of balance function measures, whereas the generic group showed significant improvement only in standing balance tests.

Cohen (1994) evaluated the benefits of intensive outpatient therapy versus a generic home-based exercise program. Fig. 6–1 indicates and Cohen's article states that "Preliminary data indicated that even a minimal program of simple head exercises practiced daily at home improves functional independence. Preliminary data also suggest that patients who participate in a more rigorous program at an outpatient clinic with an occupational therapist improve even more."

Although the concept of exercise treatment for dizziness is gaining popularity, access to VR remains limited. Yardley et al. (1998) speculate that the difficulty encountered by patients in finding VR facilities, and the time commitment required to attend regular sessions, may decrease patient compliance. They found a "much higher" rate of compliance when offering patients therapy that could be performed in their own home and speculated that the need to travel and to attend therapy sessions during working hours was a deterrent to acceptance of therapy. Blakely (1999) reports on the effectiveness of providing vestibular patients with a written list of exercises to be performed at home. The exercises were demonstrated to each patient, and then each patient was instructed to perform the exercises "two to three times in each of three to four sessions per day." Blakely (1999) reports that overall 66% of vestibular patients reported significant improvement in their symptoms after 1 month of therapy. There was no control group in this study; however, the improvement rate of 66% of patients

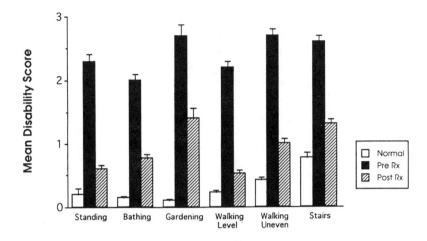

Activities of Daily Living

Figure 6–1. Level of functional disability on six activities of daily living (ADLs) for patients when healthy and before and after vestibular rehabilitation. Mean disability score is the mean of the median scores on several tasks. Rx, treatment. (Reprinted with permission from Cohen, H. (1994). Vestibular rehabilitation improves daily life function. *Am J Occup Ther*, *48*(10), 919–225.)

is consistent with Shepard and Telian's (1995, 1996) results (64%) when using generic exercises.

Adaptive Strategies

Patients with a loss of vestibular function, either unilateral or bilateral, adopt a number of strategies to increase gaze stability with head movement. In addition to the previously described recovery of the VOR through plasticity of the CNS, some behavioral changes and substitutions of vestibular responses take place.

Cervico-ocular Reflex Input

The input of the cervico-ocular reflex (COR) has been recognized since Robert Barany's work in the early 1900s. The COR is thought to be a compensatory reflexive eye movement in response to stimulation from the ligaments, muscles, and joints in the neck. The COR's input for gaze stabilization in patients with normal vestibular function is insignificant (Barlow & Freedman, 1980; Bronstein & Hood, 1986; Sawyer et al., 1994). This is probably also true of patients with unilateral vestibular loss. In patients with bilateral loss of labyrinthine function, the COR has been shown to provide a small contribution to eye–head coordination at very low speeds of head movement.

Bronstein and Hood (1986) reported that "in the absence of vestibular function, the COR appears to take on the role of the vestibulo-ocular reflex in head–eye coordination in a) the initiation of the anti-compensatory saccade which takes the eyes in the direction of the target, and b) the generation of the subsequent slow compensatory eye movements." Kasai and Zee (1978) concluded that central preprogramming played a large role in COR functioning. The COR operates only at very low frequencies in normal subjects (maximum gain at 0.025 Hz, negligible at 0.4 Hz); however, a significant contribution from the COR is noted in patients with vestibular loss up to 0.5 Hz (Barlow & Freedman, 1980; Kasai & Zee, 1978). The COR may also contribute to postural stability in normal patients because "injections of local anesthetics into the neck in humans produces temporary dysequilibrium and ataxia" (deJong, de Jong, Cohen, & Jonkees, 1977).

Modification of Saccades

Saccades are the fastest eye movements and may be voluntary or involuntary (as in the fast phase of nystagmus). Saccades allow patients to refixate their gaze with minimal duration of retinal slip. The speed of initiation of a saccade is 150 to 250 msec when the target is unpredictable and approximately 76 msec with a predictable target (Leigh & Zee, 1991). Research indicates that saccades are amenable to increased efficiency through practice. Fischer and Ramsperger (1986) report that daily practice results in a small but significant reduction in response latency and an increase in accuracy. Because response latency is significantly decreased when the target is predictable, it is likely that some central preprogramming of eye movements occurs when a patient with vestibular loss moves his or her head. These patients may make a voluntary saccade contralateral to the direction of head movement to compensate for the inefficient VOR response (Kasai & Zee, 1978). Through repetitive conditioning and feedback, patients tend to predict the necessary saccade in response to head movement. Modification of saccades is noted in patients with both unilateral and bilateral vestibular loss.

Modification of Smooth Pursuit

Smooth-pursuit tracking, or visual following, allows for gaze stability on objects moving through the field of vision. This type of eye movement is modulated by the cerebellum and can function alone while the head is still or can interact with the VOR to assist in gaze stability while moving. Smooth-pursuit tracking ability does not appear to improve in well-compensated individuals with adult-onset vestibular loss. Smooth-pursuit abilities tend to break down around 1 Hz in both normal individuals and labyrinthine-deficient patients (Gresty, Hess, & Leech, 1977; Leigh, Sharpe, Ranalli, Thurston, & Hamid, 1987). The increased plasticity of the CNS in children is evident in two reports: Chambers, Mai, and Barber (1985) report that subjects with onset of bilateral vestibular loss before adulthood did not complain of oscillopsia, whereas those with adult-onset loss did complain. Gresty et al. (1977) report on a patient with bilateral labyrinthine dysfunction since childhood demonstrating accurate smooth pursuit following up to 3 Hz.

Substitution of Sensory Inputs and Decreased Head Movements

Following the loss of vestibular function bilaterally, there is a "reweighting" of priority and dependency on visual and somatosensory inputs for the maintenance of balance and postural control (Herdman, 1994). Initially, there is a shift toward visual dependency. While walking, patients may visually lock on to targets and use this locking on to provide information about relative motion. Gradually, these patients learn to distribute more equally their dependency on proprioceptive as well as visual information.

A deficient VOR is not an issue when the head is not moving; therefore, some patients develop a strategy of avoiding any rapid head movements to avoid the symptoms of retinal slip. This strategy does not allow the natural compensation process to take place and does not alter the fact that when the head is inevitably moved quickly, symptoms will ensue.

Planning, Goal Writing, and Documentation

In establishing reasonable goals and planning a therapy program suitable for a patient, the clinician must take into consideration a number of variables, including the following:

1. A working diagnosis
2. The patient's specific complaints and concerns regarding lifestyle limitations
3. Any permanent impairments not amenable to therapy
4. A realistic expected level of improvement
5. The clinician's concerns regarding patient safety and the risk of falling

Following formal vestibular, audiologic, otologic, or neurologic evaluation, an initial pretherapy assessment will help the clinician design a specific treatment plan and will provide data for comparative outcome measures during and following therapy. The pretherapy assessment usually consists of a combination of objective and subjective tests. Objective tests may include the following:

1. Sensory organization testing. Numeric sway data can be obtained by a variety of methods and techniques including computerized platform posturography (discussed in Chapters 4 and 5).
2. Timed one-leg standing.
3. Dynamic visual acuity can be measured using a standard Snellen chart, comparing visual acuity with and without head movement (discussed in Chapter 3).

Subjective rating scales that are frequently used include the following:

1. Dizziness Handicap Inventory (DHI). The DHI (see Appendix A) consists of 25 questions designed to elicit the clinician's response to the "functional, emotional and physical impact of balance system disease" (Jacobson & Newman, 1990).

2. Motion Sensitivity Quotient (MSQ). The MSQ (see Appendix B) includes a subjective rating of the severity of symptoms related to 16 different preselected positions (Shepard & Telian, 1996).

In addition, the therapist may perform rating scales of the patient's performance during various activities.

The format for constructing an individual therapy session will seem familiar to many health care providers (HCPs). The plan for each session should include (1) objectives, (2) methods and materials, (3) results, and (4) plans for the next session (Table 6–1).

1. Objectives include a description of the activity the patient will perform, including conditions, criteria for acceptable performance, and goal and functional outcome to be achieved.
2. Methods and materials include the name of the exercise(s) to be performed, including specific conditions under which the patient is to perform (i.e., speed, time, position, range of movement). Also included would be any materials needed (e.g., physioball, mirror, targets, foam pad).
3. Results include documentation of the patient's performance, including any dizziness, nausea, or inability to perform the task to completion. This can also include a statement regarding the patient's perception of performance using a numeric rating scale. For example, no symptoms might be rated as a 1, mild symptoms as a 2, moderate symptoms as a 3, severe symptoms as a 4, and inability to perform the task at all as a 5.
4. Plans for the next session include any progression or modification of the exercises to challenge or help the patient's performance. Exercises may be discontinued, added to the patient's home program, or modified for the next session.

Each therapy session should be planned based on the results of the patient's vestibular evaluation, pretherapy assessment, and performance in the previous therapy session. Each therapy session should begin with a review of the patient's status as of the previous session and any perceived progress since that time. The clinician must be prepared to make modifications to the plan when indicated. If exercises are provoking symptoms to the point of frustration or nausea, the difficulty level may need to be reduced. If the patient can complete the exercises with no symptoms, the clinician must move on to another exercise or add another component to the exercise (e.g., standing with the eyes closed can be changed to standing with eyes closed on a compliant surface). Therapy can, and in most cases should, be performed in the home between scheduled sessions with the therapist. Frequent exercise sessions are necessary to promote learning and carryover.

The clinician must base any recommendations about home-based exercises on the patient's risk of falling. In many cases, a family member can be trained to assist the patient during exercise at home. Younger, healthier patients may not be at risk for falling and can complete most of the therapy program at home. The author's practice is to have the younger, healthy patient attend one or two in-office sessions to learn the proper technique for appropriate exercises and then have the patient return 1 or 2 weeks later to perform a therapy session while being observed by the clinician. It is not uncommon for patients to modify their exercise (usually by slowing down required movement) to avoid symptoms. The clinician then makes suggestions and appropriate additions or deletions to the therapy program. To ensure that the patient has improved satisfactorily, and to obtain outcome data, the patient is asked to attend one follow-up session several weeks later. Many patients beginning therapy, as in any exercise program, feel worse before they begin to feel better. It is my practice to ask patients to commit to 4 weeks of therapy before judging its effectiveness.

Treatment Strategies

The following are the goals of vestibular rehabilitation:

1. To minimize symptoms and functional disability
2. To increase mobility and independence
3. To reduce the risk of falls and injury

Treatment strategies are determined by the results of the vestibular evaluation, the patient's symptoms and complaints, pretherapy assessment, and the general health and physical abilities of the patient. Patients may have specific functional limitations on which they wish to focus. The patient's general health, as well as residual vestibular function, may dictate reasonable therapy goals. In designing a program for VR, it is important to keep in mind that each patient will compensate in a different way. The following exercises will assist the patient in developing compensatory strategies, but the specific compensatory technique each patient develops is unpredictable.

The following are the general guidelines for optimizing the benefits of VR:

1. Make every effort to have the patient decrease the use of centrally sedating or vestibular suppressant medications.
2. Exercises must provoke symptoms and create an "error signal." Adopt a "no pain, no gain" approach, educating the patient that the VOR will only modify its gain and symmetry when the brain recognizes a conflict or error signal situation.
3. Extensive counseling before initiating therapy may enhance patient compliance. Patients who understand their condition and its limitations and understand how their symptoms are provoked may be less fearful and more willing to continue therapy.
4. Therapy should be initiated as soon as possible. It appears that delaying therapy may not negatively affect final outcomes, but it appears to result in a longer period of therapy for similar results.
5. Therapy sessions should be performed frequently to foster carryover and motor learning.
6. Exercises should be varied in speed and direction and should simulate real-life conditions when possible.
7. Once therapy goals have been reached, a general conditioning program and maintenance exercises are necessary to prevent a return of symptoms.

8. Patients should be counseled that they may experience periods of decompensation and may require further intensive therapy.

Treatment of Unilateral Vestibular Loss

Therapy designed to treat the patient with one normal functioning labyrinth and a loss or reduction in function in the other labyrinth is frequently termed *adaptation therapy*. The following are the goals of adaptation therapy:

1. To promote tonic rebalancing of the vestibular nuclei
2. To decrease symptoms associated with head movements through habituation therapy
3. To increase gaze stability through modification and enhancement of oculomotor abilities
4. To increase postural stability through sensory integration training

Exercises to promote recovery from unilateral vestibular loss are listed in Table 6–2, and an alphabetical listing and description of each of these exercises can be found in Appendix C.

Treatment of Bilateral Vestibular Loss

Therapy designed for the patient with bilateral vestibular loss is based on the premise that there is no remaining peripheral vestibular response to head movement and therefore no VOR function. Appropriate therapy for the patient with absence of VOR function is termed *substitution therapy.*
    The following are the goals of substitution therapy:

1. To promote the use of alternative sensory inputs, such as visual and somatosensory information when vestibular function is lost
2. To promote alternative gaze stabilization strategies through enhancing oculomotor abilities and potentiating the COR
3. To teach the patient to recognize situations when alternative sensory information is unavailable or unreliable
4. To provide information regarding fall hazards and techniques to minimize the risk of falling

Exercises to promote recovery from bilateral vestibular loss are listed in Table 6–3, and a description of these exercises can be found in Appendix C.
    Another category of patients may not appear to fall into one of the two previously described groups. These patients generally have normal vestibular evaluations if evaluated by the standard test protocol that does not address VOR deficits to head speeds above the range tested by electronystagmography (ENG) and rotational chair tests. Many of these patients have unilateral vestibular hypofunction and may only demonstrate abnormalities on high-frequency rotational testing (Leigh & Brandt, 1993; Leigh, Sawyer, Grant, & Seidman, 1992). They typically do not complain of dizziness, vertigo, or postural instability but rather a sense of visual blurring or "after-motion" with rapid head movements, particularly toward the side of a mostly compensated lesion. These

Table 6–1. Example of a "Lesson Plan" for a Vestibular Therapy Session*

Objectives	Methods	Results	Plan
While walking forward, the patient will turn his or her head from side to side and up–down to show VOR and gait stability for fall prevention.	Walking with head turns: • Bring patient to hallway • 5 min in each condition 1. Side to side 2. Up–down 3. Alternating	1. [2] Minimal dizziness, good stability. 2. [2] Moderate dizziness, good stability. 3. [4] Patient was very disoriented. Slow movement.	Patient will perform side to side and up–down only at home. Repeat alternating in next session.

*The numbers noted in the results column indicate a numeric rating of the patient's perceived performance or level of subjective symptoms associated with this particular exercise.

VOR, vestibular ocular reflex.

Table 6-2. Exercises to Promote Recovery from Unilateral Loss*

Saccades: To promote accuracy and decrease latency of saccadic eye movements

Tracking: To promote smooth pursuit tracking ability and increase dynamic visual acuity with moving objects

Head movements: To promote habituation and (VOR) stability

Head movements with targets: To promote visual suppression of the VOR through a combination of saccadic and smooth-pursuit tracking

Focus head turns: To modify VOR gain and increase the stability of the VOR

Focus head turns × 2: To modify VOR gain and promote VOR stability and interaction with the smooth-pursuit system

Ankle sways: To promote the appropriate use of ankle strategy for fall prevention, increase the limits of stability (LOS), increase leg strength, and increase translational VOR stability and center of gravity (COG) control

Circle sways: Same as ankle sways

Balance-ball bounce: To promote vertical VOR stability and hip strategy

Balance board: To promote the proper use of ankle and hip strategies for fall prevention; to increase awareness of proprioceptive input; to increase VOR stability and COG control

Ball circles: To promote VOR stability; postural stability and habituation

Ball kick: To promote eye-foot coordination; COG training for fall prevention (weight shifting) and visual tracking ability

Ball toss: To promote eye-hand coordination; COG training and visual tracking

Bend and reach: To promote VOR stability and habituation to vertical movements

Ball sitting: To promote vertical VOR stability and proper use of hip strategy

Crossover step: To promote gait control and one-legged balance for walking or climbing stairs

Face to knee: To promote habituation of movement and position induced vertigo

Foam walk: To promote gait control on an uneven surface

Obstacle course: To promote gait stability in real life situations

Roll against wall: To promote VOR stability and habituation

Sit to stand: To promote habituation of movement related dizziness; increase VOR stability and leg strength.

Standing: To promote static postural stability and COG control

Trampoline ankle sway: To promote use of ankle strategy on a compliant or uneven surface

Trampoline circle sway: Same as above

Trampoline walk: To promote gait stability on a compliant or uneven surface

Walk stop: To promote gait stability and standing balance when walking is interrupted

Walking with head turns: To promote habituation, VOR stability, sensory integration, and gait stability

Walking turns: To promote habituation, VOR stability, and gait stability

---

*See Appendix C for specific instructions regarding exercise techniques.

patients are felt to have achieved a large degree of central adaptation and compensation, but they have not developed optimal alternative gaze stabilizing strategies. Exercises geared toward reducing symptoms in these patients are referred to as *gaze stabilization exercises* or eye-head coordination exercises. These exercises (Table 6-4) are also useful for patients with confirmed unilateral or

Table 6–3. Exercises to Promote Recovery from Bilateral Vestibular Loss* **

Walk stop: See Table 6–2
Ankle sways: See Table 6–2
Balance board: See Table 6–2
Balance beam: To promote increase in awareness of proprioceptive input and use of hip
    strategy
Ball circles: See Table 6–2
Ball toss and kick: See Table 6–2
Bend and reach: See Table 6–2
Crossover step: See Table 6–2
Foam walk: See Table 6–2
Imaginary targets: To potentiate the cervicoocular reflex.
Head movements: See Table 6–2
Moving saccades: To promote alternative gaze stability strategies.
Standing: See Table 6–2
Obstacle course: See Table 6–2
One-leg stand: To promote postural stability through weight shifting.
Roll against wall: See Table 6–2
Sit to stand: See Table 6–2
Stepping patterns: To promote eye–foot coordination and one legged standing.
Trace the alphabet: Same as above
Targets: See Table 6–2
Walking with head turns: See Table 6–2
Walking turns: See Table 6–2

*See Appendix C for specific instructions regarding exercise techniques.
**Some exercises used to improve VOR function in unilateral vestibular loss patients are also used in bilateral vestibular loss patients. The goal is to stimulate movement which challenges gaze stability to help the bilateral vestibular loss patient develop alternative gaze stabilization strategies.

bilateral vestibular loss as well as patients with resolved BPPV but complaining of residual dysequilibrium.

The exercises listed in Tables 6–2, 6–3, and 6–4 and described in Appendix C are a combination of exercises used in the VR programs at the American Institute of Balance (St. Petersburg, FL), University of Michigan Vestibular Laboratory, Johns Hopkins University Hospital, and those modified and developed at our VR facility.

Outcome Measures and Discharge Criteria

Currently, no standardized outcome measure can accurately state that a patient has returned to normal performance or that the patient has received maximal benefit from therapy. Outcome measures fall into two general categories: objective physical performance measures and self-report measures. Objective physical performance measures would include such things as demonstrating increased gain on rotational testing, increased visual acuity with head movement,

Table 6–4. Exercises to Promote Gaze Stability*

Hand to hand ball toss: See Table 6– 2

Saccades: See Table 6– 2
Tracking: See Table 6– 2
Head movements: See Table 6– 2
Targets: See Table 6– 2
Focus head turns: See Table 6– 2
Head circles: See Table 6– 2
Moving saccades: See Table 6– 2
Imaginary targets: See Table 6– 2
Ball circles: See Table 6– 2
Ball toss and kick: See Table 6– 2
Gait with head moves: To promote VOR and gait stability
Balance-ball bounce: See Table 6– 2
Crossover steps: See Table 6– 2

*See Appendix C for specific instructions regarding test techniques.

or improved postural stability on posturography. Although it is tempting to use these hard data to demonstrate the benefits and justify the effectiveness of vestibular therapy, these measures may or may not correlate well with improved functional performance in real life (Clendaniel, 2000). Self-report measures, although subjective, address specifically the most important issue, the patient's symptoms. The decision to discharge a patient from therapy should be based on the completion of goals set at the initial session and on the patients self-report of improvement in functional ability.

The data obtained in the pretherapy assessment are crucial in obtaining outcome measures. These objective and subjective measures can be obtained during and after the course of therapy and comparisons can be made. Cowand, Wrisley, Walker, Strasnick, & Jacobson (1998) recently reported that VR provided significant improvement in the functional and physical subtests of the DHI but did not significantly alter the emotional subtest scores. Videotaping all therapy sessions not only provides documentation of therapy activities but can also dramatically demonstrate improvement (if any) when, at the end of the therapy program, the therapist allows the patient to view comparatively their performance on specific tasks both before and after therapy.

Limits of Vestibular Rehabilitation

In designing a vestibular therapy program, the clinician must keep in mind that balance is a multisensory function, and impairments in any of the sensory systems involved in balance can limit the potential benefits of VR. As noted in the section on dynamic symptoms, there is a permanent impairment in the VOR response to rapid head movements in the direction of the damaged labyrinth. Fetter and Zee (1988) report that years after labyrinthectomy, horizontal VOR gain to rapid impulsive head movement toward the lesioned side remains significantly less than normal. At head speeds greater than 2 Hz, there are no efficient strategies for correcting retinal slip and in many well-compensated patients, this accounts for their only lasting complaint.

Unstable Lesions

Unstable lesions do not respond well to VR. Unstable lesions include conditions such as Meniere's disease and perilymph fistula. CNS adaptation is dependent on a stable asymmetry in the vestibular nuclei (Herdman, 1997). VR may be helpful in Meniere's patients if their episodes are infrequent (i.e., a minimum of several weeks between episodes), but intensive therapy would need to be reinstituted after each episode (Shepard & Telian, 1996). Ablative procedures are sometimes recommended to create a stable asymmetry. In these cases, VR should be started as soon as possible following the procedure.

Cerebellar Dysfunction

Cerebellar dysfunction as the result of stroke or degeneration inhibits VR. Tonic rebalancing and modifications to the gain of the VOR are believed to be dependent on plasticity within the cerebellum. If the cerebellum is dysfunctional, the adaptation process may be slower and limited. CNS abnormalities (e.g., cerebrovascular accident) do not necessarily inhibit vestibular compensation if the lesion is not located within the vestibular pathways, although historically these patients require longer therapy programs. It is important to keep in mind that cerebellar dysfunction can be caused by vestibular or centrally sedating medications because the goal of these medications is to reduce the asymmetry in activity by inhibiting the cerebellar response and activity within the vestibular nuclei. It is this same asymmetry that serves as a stimulus for adaptation and compensation.

Vestibular Therapy and "Central" Lesions

Patients with persistent complaints about postural stability of "central" etiology have long been considered to have limited potential benefit from vestibular therapy and have been eliminated from most studies of VR. Because the actual process of adaptation is believed to take place in the cerebellum and brainstem, injuries to the central region might reasonably limit vestibular adaptation and ultimately impair overall compensation from vestibular injury.

Cass, Borello-France, and Furman (1996) demonstrated significant improvement in postural stability following customized vestibular therapy in patients exhibiting a "vestibular loss" pattern on SOT. Patients who exhibit a "nonspecific" pattern on SOT, most of whom had previously been classified as having "central vestibular dysfunction," did not demonstrate significant improvement after similar vestibular therapy.

Conversely, Fiebert and Brown (1979) report that patients suffering from recent cerebral vascular accidents (CVA) demonstrated greater ability to ambulate following a 2-week program of vestibular stimulation than did CVA patients not receiving this program. Shepard, Telian, and Smith-Wheelock (1993) report on an observational study indicating that, whereas patients with central or mixed central peripheral lesions require longer periods of vestibular therapy, their prognosis for improvement is good. Gill-Body, Popat, Parker, and Krebs (1997) report two case studies of the effects of VR on patients with confirmed cerebellar lesions. After a 6-week course of vestibular therapy, both patients exhibited increased performance in postural and gaze stability and in self-perception of balance.

Visual, Musculoskeletal, and Cognitive Deficits

Decreases in visual acuity and decreases in strength and sensation of the lower extremities are not uncommon in the older population. The potential, then, for sensory substitution is limited if a patient has decreased vision or proprioception. Normal vision changes with aging include reduced night vision secondary to yellowing of the cornea and a slowing of pupillary reaction to lighting changes (Tideiksaar, 1989). Binocular vision plays a role in depth perception and visual feedback of relative motion. Patients with monocular or asymmetric vision are not uncommon, particularly those in the process of having cataract surgery. Patients relying on visual feedback can be hampered by bifocal lenses. It is well known that magnifying lenses induce changes in VOR gain. The patient when looking through different lenses experiences a change in magnification, which can lead to oscillopsia and visual disturbance (Demer, Porter, Goldberg, Jenkins, & Schmidt, 1989). The constant alterations in spectacle magnification experienced with use of bifocals may inhibit appropriate changes in VOR gain. Herdman (personal communication) points out that normal patients will exhibit different VOR gains for different distances and that the wearing of bifocals may present no problem for many vestibular patients. To maximize recovery of the VOR, a visual stimulus for retinal slip is needed. Patients who are visually impaired, may not be able to adequately see targets during therapy. Visual deprivation has been demonstrated to impede recovery of horizontal VOR function (Fetter & Zee, 1988). Admittedly, these patients most likely do not relate visual blurring only in response to head movements.

Patients with peripheral sensory neuropathy or decreased leg strength secondary to injury may have limited use of proprioceptive feedback. Muscular control of movements is an integral part of good balance. When strength, range of motion, and endurance are impaired, balance will eventually suffer. Specific musculoskeletal weaknesses are associated with specific balance difficulties. Muscle mass is reduced by as much as 50% in older people, and leg strength is necessary for efficient use of ankle strategy (Tideiksaar, 1989). Allison (1995) reports that decreased ankle dorsiflexion will decrease the forward limits of stability, and weakness in the hip extensors and abductors will compromise successful hip strategies used for maintenance of balance. Patients with known musculoskeletal weaknesses are candidates for conditioning and strengthening exercises; however, therapy must take these weaknesses into consideration.

Cognitive deficits related to age or head injury present obstacles to successful therapy. Many of these patients may have functional impairment beyond simple balance or vestibular deficits. Shepard and Telian (1995) recommend that vestibular therapy be used as an adjunct to a comprehensive, multidisciplinary head injury program. Minimally, patients who cannot follow instructions for vestibular therapy exercises will undoubtedly have compromised benefit.

Patient Compliance

Patient compliance is the key to a successful VR program and is noted as a factor in many published studies (Hecker et al., 1974; Norre & DeWeert, 1980). Yardley et al. (1998) report that only 2% of a group of patients considering themselves to have "handicapping dizziness" were willing to undergo formal outpatient vestibular therapy. Desmond and Touchette (1998) report that 35% of patients for whom VR was recommended elected not to participate in a therapy program. They report that most of these patients stated that they were "not interested" even though they apparently felt the need to undergo vestibular evaluation. The authors interpreted this as a lack of motivation or confidence that they could benefit from therapy. Physicians who do not understand or accept the concept of VR may reinforce this attitude. See Chapter 1 for a review of primary care management of dizziness. It is my experience that frequent phone and personal contact between patient and clinician increases compliance with vestibular therapy.

Treatment of Benign Paroxysmal Positional Vertigo

The treatment of BPPV falls in to the scope of VR as its most effective treatment involves "treatment and therapy" designed "to bring or restore to a normal or optimum state of health . . . ." (*Webster's*, 1976). The theory behind treating BPPV is unlike that of other vestibular pathologies. Whereas most VR strategies employ repetition, motor learning, and CNS plasticity in hopes of relieving symptoms, treatment for BPPV typically includes none of these. BPPV does not represent a permanent or progressive diseased state of the vestibular system. It is a mechanical dysfunction within the offending labyrinth. As a result, techniques to promote recovery from BPPV involve mechanical repair of the dysfunction rather than adaptation to the dysfunction. In fact, recent evidence regarding the pathophysiology of BPPV and the success of single treatment procedures sheds some speculation on the conclusions of many previous VR studies using BPPV patients as subjects. Some researchers (Hecker et al., 1974; Norre & DeWeert, 1980) concluded that patients with positional vertigo improved as a result of habituation and adaptive plasticity. More recent findings regarding the natural remitting course of BPPV and the speed at which recent repositioning techniques result in resolution of symptoms indicate that at least some of the patients noting improvement in these earlier studies did not improve for the reasons described by the authors.

Pathophysiology of BPPV

There is general agreement that the site of lesion in BPPV is the ampulla of the offending semicircular canal, with the posterior canal of one labyrinth involved in 90% of cases (Fife, 1995).

Typical Diagnostic Signs of BPPV

1. A provoking position (lying supine with affected ear down)
2. A short latency before vertigo and nystagmus occur (usually 3 to 15 seconds)
3. Severe subjective vertigo accompanied by nystagmus (typically geotropic rotary nystagmus when the posterior canal is involved)
4. Short duration of symptoms (usually less than 1 minute)
5. Fatigability (repeated provocation results in a reduced response)
6. A reversal in the direction of nystagmus upon rising (sometimes)

Many patients with BPPV also complain of associated dysequilibrium and postural instability. Black and Nashner (1984) and Baloh, Honrubia, and Jacobson (1987) report a significant correlation between BPPV and abnormal posturography scores. There is some speculation that there may be abnormal responses from the affected semicircular canal or that the otolith structures (particularly the ipsilateral utricle) are no longer functioning symmetrically as a result of displaced otoconia. Additionally, there is a high incidence (32 to 47%) of abnormal caloric responses in patients with BPPV (Baloh et al., 1987; Norre & Beckers, 1987). Karlberg, Hall, Quickert, Hinson and Halmagyi (2000) report that 3% of a large group of patients with confirmed BPPV ($n = 2847$) had additional vestibulopathy in the same ear as the BPPV. The most common ipsilateral pathology was noted to be vestibular neuritis/labyrinthitis; the second most common was Meniere's disease.

Schuknecht (1969) first proposed the *theory of cupulolithiasis* in which he suggested that BPPV was the result of otoconial debris attached to the cupula of the offending posterior semicircular canal. Epley (1992) offered an alternative *theory of canalithiasis*, which more thoroughly explains the source of the above mentioned typical signs and symptoms of BPPV. The theory of canalithiasis proposes that there are free-floating particles (otoconia) which have gravitated from the utricle and collect near the cupula of the posterior canal. When the head is moved into a position that causes the particles to move away from the cupula, the resulting hydrodynamic drag causes cupular deflection (and asymmetric stimulation) resulting in vertigo and nystagmus until the particles come to rest in the now gravitationally dependent section of the canal. It is likely that both of these conditions exist (Herdman, Tusa, Zee, Proctor, & Mattox, 1993; Steddin & Brandt, 1996) and treatments have been proposed for both.

Treatment for Cupulolithiasis

As noted earlier, Brandt and Daroff (1980) found that the symptoms of BPPV were quickly relieved by repeatedly provoking symptoms through head positioning exercises. They speculated that the noted rapid improvement was not a result of habituation, but rather a means of "dispersion of otolithic debri from the cupula." Toupet and Semont (1985) took this a step further and proposed the first single treatment approach for BPPV. Norre and Beckers (1987) report that this "brisk method" effectively resolved the symptoms of BPPV in 52% of patients within one week. Currently known as the *Liberatory* or *Semont* maneuver, it was described in detail by Semont, Freyss, and Vitte (1988) (Fig. 6–2). Semont and his colleagues, over an eight year period involving 711 cases, report an 84% success rate following one maneuver and a 93% success rate following two maneuvers. More recently, Serefini, Palmieri, and Simoncelli (1996) report that complete resolution of symptoms was achieved within one treatment in more than 50% of cases; while more than 90% of cases were resolved within five treatment sessions. Theoretically, the movement required to displace otoconia from the cupula must be relatively rapid, and may be contraindicated in elderly patients or patients with a history of back or neck problems.

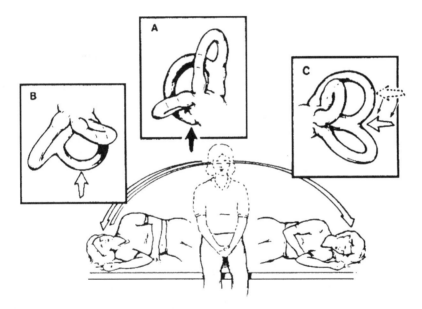

Figure 6–2. The Semont maneuver: The patient is moved quickly from sitting (A) into the position that provokes vertigo (B) and is kept in that position for 2 to 3 minutes. She is then turned rapidly to the opposite ear-down position (C), with the therapist maintaining the alignment of the neck and head on the body. The patient must stay in this position for 5 minutes. The patient is then slowly taken into a seated position. She must remain in the vertical position for 48 hours and avoid the provoking position for 1 week. The position of the right labyrinth is shown in each head position, and the posterior canal is shaded. The solid arrow indicates the location of the cupula of the posterior canal; the open arrow indicates the location of debris free-floating in the long arm of the posterior canal during the different stages of the treatment. (Reprinted with permission from Herdman, S. J., Tusa, R. J., Zee, D. S., Proctor, L. R., & Mattox, D. E. (1993). Single treatment approaches to benign paroxysmal positional vertigo. *Arch Otolaryngol Head Neck Surg*, *119*, 450–454.)

Treatment for Canalithiasis

The canalith repositioning procedure for canalithiasis was introduced by Dr. John Epley of the Portland Otologic Clinic (Epley & Hughes, 1980). This procedure has undergone several modifications and is known by a variety of names:

1. CRP (canalith repositioning procedure)
2. CRM (canalith repositioning maneuver)
3. Particle repositioning maneuver
4. Epley maneuver

All these procedures are based on the belief that free-floating otoconia in the posterior canal are responsible for BPPV. The goal of each maneuver is to cause the otoconia debris to migrate out of the posterior canal, through the common crus, and into the vestibule (Fig. 6–3). Yamane, Imoto, Nakai, Igarashi, and Rask-Anderson (1984) propose that "dark cells" of the utricle absorb and dissolve the otoconia, whereas others (Mira, Valli, Zucca, & Valli, 1996) suggest that the otoconia harmlessly dissolve in the endolymph. This issue is unresolved at this time.

The efficacy of canalith repositioning procedures has been detailed in a number of studies, with success rates typically around 90% (Desmond & Touchette, 1998; Epley, 1992; Lynn, Pool, Rose, Brey, & Suman, 1995; Parnes & Robichaud, 1997). Lynn et al. (1995) performed CRP on one group of patients with BPPV and a "placebo" procedure on a second group. Eighty-nine percent of those treated with CRP were symptom free 1 month after treatment, whereas 27% treated with the "placebo" procedure were improved. The natural course of BPPV, with frequent spontaneous remission within a few weeks, may be a confounding factor in determining precisely the success rate of CRP. Steenerson and Cronin (1996) compared the relative efficacy of vestibular habituation therapy and CRP. They found that after 3 months, 63% of patients treated with habituation therapy were symptom free, whereas 82% treated with CRP were symptom free. Only 25% of a control group receiving no treatment reported resolution of symptoms. Additionally, these authors suggest that CRP results in faster resolution of symptoms and may be better tolerated by patients than habituation therapy, which repeatedly provokes symptoms.

Epley's (1992) original description of the CRP is as follows:

1. Preliminary—Identification of offending canal and noted latency and duration of nystagmus response
2. Preparation—Premedication with transdermal scopolamine or diazepam
3. Maneuvers—Commencement of maneuvers as described in Fig. 6–3, changing head positions when the nystagmus response has ceased. If no nystagmus is appreciated, then an estimate of latency plus duration of previous response (typically "6 to 13 seconds") dictates when the head is moved to the next position. Complete cycles are performed until there is no nystagmus response.
4. Oscillation—A hand-held oscillator with a frequency of approximately 80 Hz is applied to the mastoid process of the affected side.

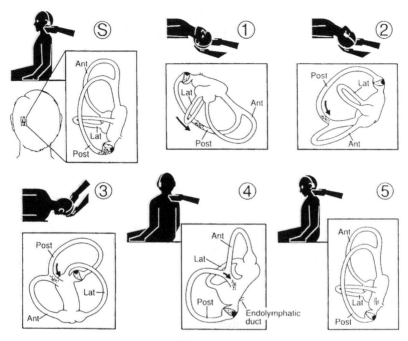

Figure 6–3. Canalith repositioning procedure: Positions of the left posterior semicircular canal (PSC). Sitting (1) Patient is brought into the offending left Hallpike position, causing flow of debris away from cupula of the left PSC. (2) While the patient remains in the supine position, the patient's head is rotated to the right side. (3) With the orientation of the head to the right shoulder unchanged, the patient is rolled over onto the right shoulder and hip, looking down toward the floor. (4) The head remains to the right, tilted down, and the patient rises to the sitting position. (5) The head is rotated forward, chin tilted down. *Note:* The patient should be kept in each of these positions until nystagmus has ceased or for a period at least equal to the duration of time from initiating the provoking (Hallpike) maneuver to the cessation of nystagmus. Nystagmus should be viewed in all positions because a change in the direction of nystagmus indicates possible failure to deposit all of the debris in the vestibule. (Reprinted and adapted with permission from Epley, J. (1992). The canalith repositioning procedure: for treatment of benign paroxysmal positional vertigo. *Otolaryngol Head Neck Surg*, *107*(3), 399–404.)

5. Follow-up—Patients are advised to keep their head upright for 48 hours following the procedure. The CRP may be repeated weekly until the patient is asymptomatic and no nystagmus is noted in the Hallpike position (Epley, 1992).

Subsequent reports have offered modifications of the CRP. Many investigators and practicing clinicians do not use any type of oscillation (Herdman et al., 1993; Parnes & Robichaud, 1997; Steenerson & Cronin, 1996) and have reported results similar to those of Epley (1992). Li (1995) noted a significantly reduced rate of resolution of symptoms following one treatment with CRP in patients not treated with oscillation during the procedure.

The length of time that the patient needs to remain upright following treatment has also been modified. Some time is recommended to keep the free-floating otoconia from gravitating back into the posterior canal. Whereas most published reports recommend 48 hours, Herdman (2001) advocates the use of a soft neck collar and that the patient remain upright for only 24 hours following treatment. Many patients are reluctant to spend a night sitting up in a chair. For these patients, I have performed the CRP early in the morning and asked the patient to remain upright as long as possible. My experience has been that this technique is quite effective both in obtaining consent for the procedure and in resolving symptoms in most patients. This is recommended only if the patient objects to the standard follow-up period.

More recent publications indicate that both the Semont maneuver and the CRP are effective in treating either form of BPPV (Parnes & Price-Jones, 1993). Cohen and Jerabek (1999) suggest that the criteria for choosing should be based on nonotologic factors because both techniques appear to be equally effective in relieving positional vertigo. They state that the Semont maneuver can be more easily applied to patients with limited range of motion or with arthritis or neck or back problems. The CRP is preferable for large or obese patients as the clinician can more easily perform this procedure without assistance.

Finally, Herdman and Tusa (1996) caution that even with correct performance of the CRP, it is possible inadvertently to deposit the otoconia into the horizontal or anterior semicircular canals. To avoid this, they recommend that the eyes be observed carefully for direction of nystagmus during all head positions of CRP. If the direction of rotary nystagmus reverses or the nystagmus converts from a rotary to a horizontal pattern, the examiner needs to consider the possibility of conversion from posterior to horizontal or anterior canal BPPV.

Variant Forms of Benign Paroxysmal Positional Vertigo

In the last several years, BPPV of the anterior and horizontal semicircular canals has been reported (Fife, 1995; Lempert & Tiel-Wick, 1996; Stockwell, 1996). Fife (1995) estimates that anterior canal BPPV accounts for 4% of all cases, with horizontal canal involvement in 6% of cases. The remaining 90% are believed to involve the posterior canal. Both canalithiasis and cupulolithiasis have been implicated as causative factors and may be determining factors in the direction of nystagmus noted. Anterior canal BPPV is most typically provoked by a Hallpike maneuver with the affected ear on the up side. Because the same position can trigger posterior canal BPPV of the down side ear, differentiating canal involvement is done by observing the direction of nystagmus while the patient experiences vertigo. As noted earlier, posterior canal BPPV is marked by *geotropic* (beating toward the earth) and upbeating rotary nystagmus; in anterior canal BPPV, the nystagmus is primarily *ageotropic* (beating away from the earth) and downbeating (Stockwell, 1996). Treatment of anterior canal BPPV may be accomplished by performing CRP as though treating posterior canal BPPV in the opposite ear. Herdman and Tusa (1999) recommend a modification of the Semont maneuver to treat anterior canal BPPV.

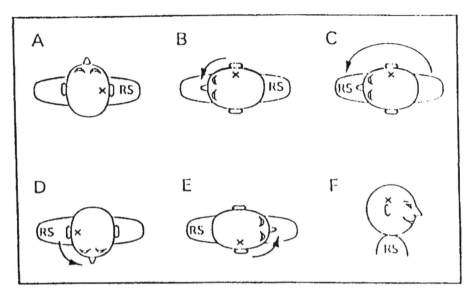

Figure 6–4. Positional maneuver for treatment of horizontal canal benign paroxysmal positional vertigo. Each 90-degree head rotation is performed rapidly within a half second. Head positions are maintained for between 30 and 60 seconds until all nystagmus has subsided. (A) Starting position; supine. (B) Head rotation toward the unaffected ear. (C) Body turn from supine to prone while head positions are maintained. (D) Head rotation to nose-down position. (E) Final head turn to affected-ear-down position. (F) Sitting-up position. X , affected ear (right side); RS, right shoulder. (Reprinted with permission from Lempert, T., & Tiel-Wilck, K. (1996). Positional maneuver for treatment of horizontal-canal benign positional vertigo. *Laryngoscope, 106*, 476–478.)

Horizontal canal BPPV may be elicited during the Hallpike maneuver but is best provoked by having the patient lie flat in the supine position and then move the head quickly to the ear down position, both to the right and the left. Horizontal canal BPPV (canalithiasis) may be diagnosed by observing horizontal geotropic nystagmus with no rotary component while the patient is vertiginous. The patient is typically more vertiginous and the intensity of the nystagmus greater when the affected ear is down. As in other forms of BPPV, there is a short latency and a transient response with a duration typically longer than that observed in BPPV of the other two canals. Repositioning technique for horizontal canal BPPV involves having the patient start in the supine position and then rotate 360 degrees in the direction away from the affected canal (Fig. 6–4).

Baloh (1996) describes horizontal canal cupulolithiasis where it is speculated that otolith debris attaches to the cupula of the horizontal semicircular canal. When the patient rolls toward the affected side, the debris causes an abnormal weighting of the cupula away from the utricle (Fig. 6–5). Nystagmus beating away from the downside ear is noted. When the patient rolls away from the affected ear onto the unaffected ear, the nystagmus reverses as a result of the cupula on the upside ear being abnormally weighted toward the utricle. Baloh

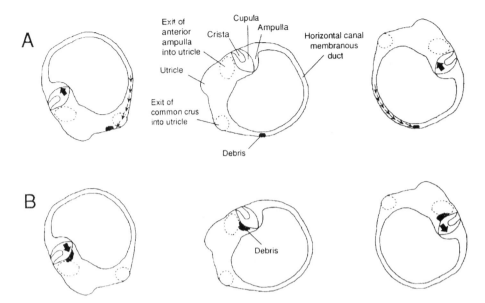

Figure 6–5. Proposed mechanisms of paroxysmal (A) and persistent (B) horizontal canal positional nystagmus. With the paroxysmal variant (A) the debris is freely moving within the canal; with the persistent variant (B) the debris is attached to the cupula. The positioning of the utricle and ampulla relative to the head was derived from computed tomography scans of normal human temporal bones with cuts through the horizontal semicircular canal. Small arrows indicate movement of debris within the endolymph. Large arrows indicate the direction of cupula deviation. (Reprinted with permission from Baloh, R. (1996). Benign positional vertigo. In R. Baloh, & G. M. Halmagyi (Eds.), *Disorders of the vestibular system* (pp.328–339). New York: Oxford University Press)

(1996) suggests that provocation exercises used for posterior canal BPPV may dislodge the debris and seemed to work for one patient presenting with the above-described pattern of nystagmus.

Although success rates of CRP are impressive, some patients with intractable positional vertigo will not respond to repositioning procedures. These patients may be candidates for surgical intervention. Surgical procedures to relieve the symptoms of BPPV include sectioning of the posterior nerve (singular neurectomy) to eliminate the response from the ampulla of the posterior canal and occlusion of the posterior canal (canal plugging) to preclude loose otoconia from entering the posterior canal (Gacek, 1991; Parnes & McClure, 1990).

Home Treatment of Benign Paroxysmal Positional Vertigo

Some patients will have a history consistent with BPPV; however, Hallpike tests on the day of examination fail to provoke an episode of vertigo and rescheduling may be necessary (see Chapter 5 for details). If an episode of BPPV can be provoked at a later date, appropriate repositioning can be completed. Occasionally, a patient will not be willing or able to return or may have a negative

Hallpike test a second or third time. In these instances, home-based exercises may be recommended.

Brandt–Daroff Exercises

Home provocation exercises intended to relieve BPPV have been used since they were introduced by Brandt and Daroff in 1980. Prior to 1980, many patients with symptoms of BPPV were advised to avoid the offending position. Brandt and Daroff (1980) speculated that repeated provocation of the positional vertigo would "promote loosening and ultimate dispersion of the otolithic debris from the cupula." They reported that 66 of 67 patients "experienced complete relief of the positional vertigo within 14 days, with most requiring 7 to 10 days. Positional nystagmus was absent too." The Brandt–Daroff exercises (BDE) as described in Fig. 6–6 are designed to provoke intentionally episodes of BPPV repeatedly in a controlled, safe manner. The positions (and accompanying figure) are strikingly similar to those used in the Semont maneuver (discussed earlier in this chapter). The movements differ in that in the BDEs the patient comes back to the sitting position and rests before continuing with additional movements. If the offending ear has been identified, the BDEs can be performed in the direction of the offending side only.

In our clinic, I modified the BDE by having the patient perform the Hallpike maneuver while lying in bed. I have the patient place a pillow under the shoulder blades to allow the offending otoliths to move farther along the posterior canal.

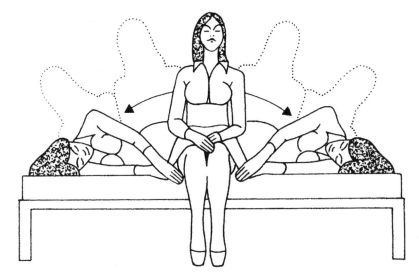

Figure 6–6. Brandt and Daroff's exercise for benign paroxysmal positional vertigo is performed by having the patient repeatedly move from sitting to the affected side, waiting until the vertigo stops and then resuming the sitting position. The movement can then be repeated in the opposite direction if the affected side is unknown. (Reprinted with permission from Brandt, T., & Daroff, R. (1980). Physical therapy for benign paroxysmal positional vertigo. *Arch Otolaryngol, 106, 484–485.*)

After the vertigo has ceased, or 1 minute has passed, the patient is instructed to sit up quickly, hoping that some of the dispersed otoliths will migrate toward the common crus and out of the posterior canal. Theoretically, with repeated provocation, enough otoliths will be dispersed from the posterior canal to reduce or eliminate the pathologic condition. This modification has not undergone any controlled studies and is speculative as to whether it is more efficient than the BDE technique. I recently switched to the exercises described by Radtke, Neuhauser, von Brevern, and Lempert (1999) described as follows.

Modified Epley Procedure

Radtke et al. (1999) compared the efficacy of BDE to a modified canalith-repositioning procedure intended for self-treatment of BPPV (Figs. 6–7 and 6–8).

Self-treatment of benign positional vertigo (right)

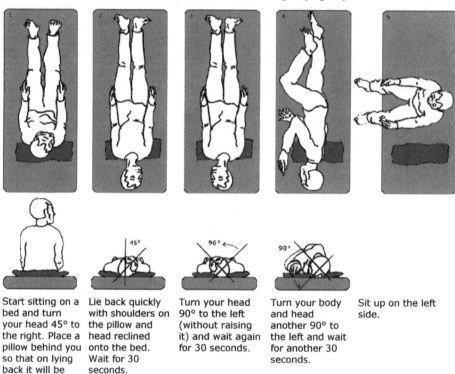

| Start sitting on a bed and turn your head 45° to the right. Place a pillow behind you so that on lying back it will be under your shoulders. | Lie back quickly with shoulders on the pillow and head reclined onto the bed. Wait for 30 seconds. | Turn your head 90° to the left (without raising it) and wait again for 30 seconds. | Turn your body and head another 90° to the left and wait for another 30 seconds. | Sit up on the left side. |

This maneuver should be carried out three times a day. Repeat this daily until you are free from positional vertigo for 24 hours.

Figure 6–7. Right self-treatment technique. (Reprinted with permission from Radtke, A., Neuhauser, H., von Brevern, M., & Lempert, T. (1999). A modified Epley's procedure for self-treatment of benign paroxysmal positional vertigo. *Neurology, 53,* 1358–1360.)

Self-treatment of benign positional vertigo (left)

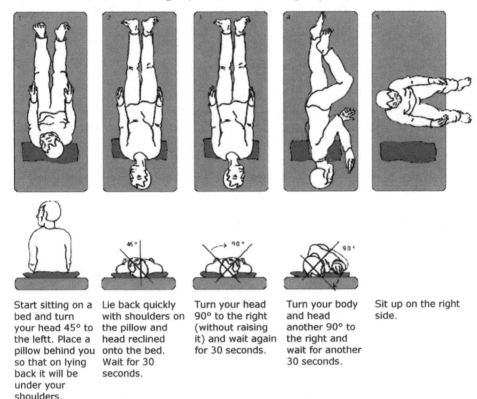

Start sitting on a bed and turn your head 45° to the leftt. Place a pillow behind you so that on lying back it will be under your shoulders.	Lie back quickly with shoulders on the pillow and head reclined onto the bed. Wait for 30 seconds.	Turn your head 90° to the right (without raising it) and wait again for 30 seconds.	Turn your body and head another 90° to the right and wait for another 30 seconds.	Sit up on the right side.

This maneuver should be carried out three times a day. Repeat this daily until you are free from positional vertigo for 24 hours.

Figure 6–8. Left self-treatment technique. (Reprinted with permission from Radtke, A., Neuhauser, H., von Brevern, M., & Lempert, T. (1999). A modified Epley's procedure for self-treatment of benign paroxysmal positional vertigo. *Neurology, 53,* 1358–1360.)

Their "modified Epley procedure" (MEP) is similar to the previously described repositioning procedure described by Epley with the exceptions of no oscillation, no antiemetic medication, and no follow-up period of keeping the head erect after repositioning. Patients are instructed to perform the modified procedure three times a day each day until they are free from positional vertigo for 24 hours. Radtke et al. (1999) report that "after one week, 18 of 28 (64%) using the MEP were asymptomatic compared with 6 of 26 patients (23%) using the BDE." While these data indicate that the MEP may be more effective than the BDE, neither is nearly as effective as single-treatment CRP as described earlier.

Research and clinical experience indicate that a large number of patients suffering from vestibular dysfunction can benefit from vestibular therapy. Past approaches to treating dizzy patients have been shown to be less effective than a customized intensive therapy program. Acceptance of VR is still in its early stages, however. The goal of this chapter is to review the clinical evidence, explain the basis for vestibular adaptation and compensation, and give the reader some practical tools to begin a VR program.

Prevention of Falls

Even with VR, patients with vestibular loss are at higher risk for falling, particularly in situations where visual and somatosensory information is absent or unreliable. Falls are one of the most serious problems associated with aging. The statistics are startling. It is estimated that one third to one half of all people over 65 years of age fall at least once (Coogler, 1992). In fact, falls are the leading cause of injury in older adults and account for more than 200,000 hip fractures annually in the United States alone (Haupt & Graves, 1982). Of these, 25% will never regain full mobility (Coogler, 1992). In essence, a fall leading to a hip fracture can forever change a patient's life.

From the perspective of the older patient, these statistics make it clear that fall prevention programs are important and worthwhile. HCPs also need to recognize that fall prevention planning can significantly reduce health care costs. The cost of direct care alone for hip fracture patients is in the billions of dollars annually (Allison, undated). Additionally, many of these patients are admitted to chronic care institutions (Tinetti & Williams, 1997).

Numerous factors contribute to putting one at a higher risk for falling. A variety of medical conditions, including peripheral neuropathy, postural hypotension, and transient ischemic attacks may contribute to an increased risk for falling. Among the most common reasons are decreased efficiency of the systems (visual, vestibular, and proprioceptive) that send information regarding balance and movement to the brain.

Older people, as we know, lose visual acuity. In addition, they require more light to see clearly while at the same time having a reduced tolerance for glare. Older people also require more time to adjust to lighting changes. This means that their visual world is not as predictable or useful in helping maintain balance as it would be for someone with normal vision.

Older people also have lengthened reaction time in many situations. When younger, healthy people stumble or slip, they can react quickly and "catch" themselves in time. Older people often do not react until they have reached a point that exceeds their limits of stability (defined in Chapter 2).

Muscle mass and strength decrease with age. To maintain balance or to recover from a loss of balance, we must have sufficient strength in our legs to push us back to an upright position. Additionally, many older people with circulatory problems have reduced sensation or feeling in their lower legs, causing their physical contact with the world to be unreliable and less useful when they are standing.

As mentioned earlier in the section on the limits of VR, some patients with vestibular loss may be susceptible to falling under certain conditions. For these patients, education as to potential fall hazards and environmental modifications to minimize fall hazards is indicated. For a thorough review of fall prevention environmental assessments and appropriate modifications, the reader is referred to *Falling in Old Age: Its Prevention and Treatment* (Tideiksaar, 1989).

Medical/ Surgical Treatment Options

Medical Treatment of the Dizzy Patient

Although there is general agreement among specialists in the area of VR that vestibular compensation is inhibited by the use of vestibular or CNS sedative medications (Brandt, 1991; Shepard et al., 1990; Zee, 1985), the literature suggests that these types of medications are used most of the time when a patient presents in the primary care setting with a complaint of dizziness, vertigo, or imbalance (Sloane et al., 1994; Burke, 1995). Medical treatment falls into two broad categories: those in which the symptoms are treated, as mentioned previously, and those used in hopes of controlling the underlying pathologic condition responsible for these complaints.

Vestibular Suppressants

Medication used to suppress symptoms would ideally be used only during the acute stage following vestibular insult. Appropriate treatment following the acute phase would include activity to promote adaptation and compensation. Additionally, some patients describing imbalance may have perfectly normal vestibular function and may be experiencing imbalance or dysequilibrium from another cause. These patients may actually experience greater symptoms because suppressant medications may hinder the function of the vestibular apparatus at a time when the patient may be most dependent on it.

The most common sedative or suppressant medications include meclizine (Antivert) and dimenhydrinate (Dramamine). These antihistamines are used to reduce the sensation of vertigo and accompanying nausea by reducing the activity in the vestibular nuclei. Side effects are drowsiness and CNS depression. Phenothiazines such as promethazine (Phenergan) and prochlorperazine (Compazine) are primarily used to treat nausea frequently associated with acute vertigo. Sedatives such as diazepam (Valium) also reduce activity within the vestibular nuclei, as well as treat the patient's anxiety reaction. Sedatives also cause CNS depression and may be habit forming.

Prophylactic Medications

Medications used to treat underlying pathology are primarily prophylactic. Because the most common vestibular disease causing recurrent episodes of unprovoked vertigo is Meniere's disease, most medications in this group are chosen based on the treating physician's belief in the pathophysiology of Meniere's disease. The variety of treatments for Meniere's disease reflects the lack of definitive evidence of efficacy for any one treatment. Most commonly, attempts at reducing endolymphatic pressure are used. Patients are placed on a low-salt diet and often treated with diuretics, most frequently HCTZ or Dyazide.

Although there is little conclusive evidence that diuretics are effective in treating Meniere's disease, van Deelen and Huizing (1986) reported a significant reduction in complaints of vertigo in Meniere's patients using Dyazide. In addition to a low-salt diet, patients are often instructed to avoid CATS: caffeine, alcohol, tobacco, and stress (Arenberg, 1993).

Vasodilators such as nicotinic acid or Hydergine are sometimes prescribed in hopes of increasing blood flow to the labyrinth and brain stem. This treatment is based on the belief that Meniere's disease is a result of ischemia of the stria vascularis. There are no known studies regarding efficacy of this treatment (Moffat & Ballagh, 1997). High-dose steroids may be prescribed based on the belief that Meniere's disease is an immune system response. Diet restrictions are also advocated with this approach (Dereberry, 1989).

Surgical Treatment of Unstable Vestibular Lesions

When output from, or activity of, a single peripheral vestibular apparatus is unstable or fluctuant, lasting vestibular compensation cannot take place. The goal of surgical intervention is to create a stable vestibular end organ. Depending on the suspected source of instability, surgical approaches may be reparative or ablative.

Reparative procedures include repair of perilymphatic fistula and decompression of the endolymphatic sac. Because there is no reliable way to diagnose a perilymph fistula preoperatively and no way to verify objectively an improvement in symptoms postoperatively, the decision to explore the ear surgically is based largely the surgeon's belief in the incidence of perilymph fistula in the "dizzy" population.

Portman (1927) introduced endolymphatic sac decompression, with noted resolution of Meniere's-type symptoms. Thomsen, Bretlau, Tos, and Johnson (1981) reported their "sham study" in which they performed simple mastoidectomy with sac decompression in one group and mastoidectomy without sac decompression in a second group. Group 1 noted improvement in 73%, whereas group 2 had an improvement rate of 80%. Silverstein, Smouha, and Jones (1989) followed up on two groups of patients for more than 8 years. Group 1 had endolymphatic sac surgery; group 2 had no surgery. They noted no significant difference in reported relief of vertigo. There are many anecdotal reports of complete resolution of symptoms following endolymphatic sac surgery.

Surgical ablative procedures have historically been offered as a last resort because of the complications inherent in cranial surgery. Eighth nerve section for vertigo was introduced by R. H. Parry (1904), but it was popularized by Dandy, who performed more than 400 such procedures between 1928 and 1941 with good success. Of course, total loss of hearing on the operated side was inevitable. McKenzie (1936) refined this technique by sectioning only the vestibular nerve, with hearing preserved in most cases. Silverstein, Rosenberg, Arruda, and Isaacson (1997) report that with selective nerve section, not only can hearing be preserved, but more than two thirds of selected patients reported relief of tinnitus on the affected side. Harold Schuknecht (1957) reported that in cases where there was no preservable hearing, Labyrinthectomy provided relief of vertigo in approximately 90% of patients with recurrent vertigo. Complications of these surgical ablative procedures included prolonged instability, a small incidence of facial nerve injuries, cerebrospinal fluid leaks, and meningitis.

Chemical Ablative Procedures

Intratympanic aminoglycoside treatment for recurrent vertigo was introduced by Schuknecht in 1956. Although relief of vertigo was noted following injection of streptomycin, all patients treated in this manner suffered profound hearing loss. Shea (1989) investigated perfusion of streptomycin into the horizontal semicircular canal, followed by lower dose intramuscular injections of streptomycin. Again, an unacceptable rate of hearing loss was noted. Streptomycin used parentally has been used successfully in cases of bilateral Meniere's disease. Parental administration causes vestibular ablation (or at least enough reduction in function to eliminate vertigo) with little effect on hearing (Moffat & Ballagh, 1997).

More recently, gentamicin has been used for vestibular ablation because it has minimal cochleotoxic effects in low doses. Introduced by Beck and Schmidt (1978), intratympanic injection of gentamicin has been the subject of several reports indicating a high incidence of relief of vertigo with a relatively low incidence of hearing loss (Murofushi, Halmagyi, & Yavor, 1997; Odkvist, Bergenius, & Miller, 1997; Trine, Lynn, Facer, & Kasperbauer, 1995).

Minor (1999) describes a protocol for optimal results when using intratympanic gentamicin to control episodic vertigo associated with Meniere's disease. Candidates for gentamicin therapy must fit the Academy of Otolaryngology–Head and Neck Surgery criteria for "definite" Meniere's disease, must have serviceable hearing in the affected ear, must not have symptoms suggestive of Meniere's disease in the contralateral ear, and must not have responded to conservative medical therapy. Injections are given weekly, and the patient is assessed for residual vestibular function weekly through caloric and rotational chair studies. Weekly injections are stopped when objective evidence of vestibular hypofunction is obtained. Following this protocol, Minor reports control of vertigo in 91% of patients and profound hearing loss in 3% (one patient).

References

Allison, L. (1995). Balance disorders. In: D. A. Umphred (Ed.), *Neurological rehabilitation* (pp. 802–837), 3rd ed. St. Louis: Mosby-Year Book.

Allison, L. (undated). Identifying and managing elderly fallers. *Neurocom International Literature*, 1–8.

Arenberg, I. K. (1993). Meniere's disease: diagnosis and management of vertigo and endolymphatic hydrops. In: *Dizziness and balance disorders* (pp. 503–510). New York: Kugler Publications.

Baloh, R. (1996). Benign positional vertigo. In: R. Baloh, & G. M. Halmagyi (Eds.), *Disorders of the vestibular system* (pp. 328–339). New York: Oxford University Press.

Baloh, R., Honrubia, V., & Jacobson, K. (1987.) Benign positional vertigo: Clinical and oculographic features in 240 cases. *Neurology, 37*, 371–378.

Barlow, D., & Freedman, W. (1980). Cervico-ocular reflex in the normal adult. *Acta Otolaryngol, 89*, 487–496.

Beck, C., & Schmidt, C. (1978). Ten years of experience with intratympanally applied streptomycin (gentamicin) in the therapy of morbus Meiniere. *Arch Otolaryngol*, *221*, 149–152.

Black, F. O., & Nashner, L. M. (1984). Postural disturbances in patients with benign paroxysmal positional nystagmus. *Ann Otol Rhinol Laryngol*, *93*, 595–599.

Blakely, B. (1999). Vestibular rehabilitation on a budget. *J Otolaryngol*, *28*(4), 205–210.

Brandt, T. (1991). Medical and physical therapy. In: Brandt, T. (Ed.), *Vertigo: Its multisensory syndromes* (pp. 15–17). New York: Springer-Verlag.

Brandt, T., & Daroff, R. (1980). Physical therapy for benign paroxysmal positional vertigo. *Arch Otolaryngol*, *106*, 484–485.

Bronstein, A. M., & Hood, D. (1986). The cervico-ocular reflex in normal subjects and patients with absent vestibular function. *Brain Res*, *373*, 399–408.

Burke, M. (1995). Dizziness in the elderly: etiology and treatment. *Nurse Pract*, *20*(12), 28–35.

Cass, S. P, Borello-France, D., & Furman, J. M. (1996). Functional outcome of vestibular rehabilitation in patients with abnormal sensory-organization testing. *Am J Otol*, *17*, 581–594.

Cawthorne, T. (1945a). The physiological basis for head exercises. *J Chartered Soc Physiother*, *30*, 106–107.

Cawthorne, T. (1945b). Vestibular injuries. *Proc R Soc Med*, *39*, 270–273.

Chambers, B. R., Mai, M., & Barber, H. O. (1985). Bilateral vestibular loss, oscillopsia, and the cervico-ocular reflex. *Otolaryngol Head Neck Surg*, *93*, 403–407.

Clendaniel, R. A. (2000). Outcome measures for assessment of treatment of the dizzy and balance disorder patient. *Otolaryngol Clin North Am*, *33*(3), 519–533.

Cohen, H. (1994). Vestibular rehabilitation improves daily life function. *Am J Occup Ther*, *48*(10), 919–925.

Cohen, H., & Jerabek, J. (1999). Efficacy of treatments for posterior canal benign paroxysmal positional vertigo. *Laryngoscope*, *109*, 584–590.

Coogler, C. E. (1992, April/May). Falls and imbalance. *Rehabil Manage*, *53*.

Cooksey, F. S. (1945). Rehabilitation in vestibular injuries. *Proc R Soc Med Sect Otol*, *2*, 273–278.

Courjon, J. H., Jeannerod, M., Ossuzio, I., & Schmid, R. (1977). The role of vision in compensation of vestibulo ocular reflex after hemilabyrinthectomy in the cat. *Exp Brain Res*, *28*, 235–248.

Cowand, J., Wrisley, D., Walker, M., Strasnick, B., & Jacobson, J. (1998). Efficacy of vestibular rehabilitation. *Otolaryngol Head Neck Surg*, *118*(1), 49–54.

deJong, P. T. V. M., deJong V. J. M. B., Cohen, B., & Jonkees, L. B. W. (1977). Ataxia and nystagmus induced by injection of local anesthetics in the neck. *Ann Neurol*, *1*, 240–246.

Dereberry, J. (August 1989). Food allergies and Meniere's disease. *New Horizons in Otolaryngologic Allergy*, 1–3.

Demer, J. L., Porter, F. I., Goldberg, J., Jenkins, H. A., & Schmidt, K. (1989). Adaptation to telescopic spectacles: vestibulo-ocular reflex plasticity. *Invest Opthalmol Vis Sci*, *30*(1), 159–170.

Desmond, A. L., & Touchette, D. A. (1998). *Balance disorders: Evaluation and treatment; A short course for primary care physicians*. Micromedical Technologies. Chathan, IL.

Dix, M. (1984). Rehabilitation of vertigo. In: M. R. Dix & J. D. Hood, J. D. (Eds.), *Vertigo* (pp. 467–479). New York: John Wiley & Sons.

Epley, J. (1992). The canalith repositioning procedure: for treatment of benign paroxysmal positional vertigo. *Otolaryngol Head Neck Surg*, *107*(3), 399–404.

Epley, J., & Hughes, D. W. (1980). Positional vertigo: new methods of diagnosis and treatment. [Abstract] *Otolaryngol Head Neck Surg*, *88*, 49.

Fetter, M., & Zee, D. (1988). Recovery from unilateral labyrinthectomy in rhesus monkey. *Neurophysiology*, *59*(2), 370–393.

Fiebert, I., & Brown, E. (1979). Vestibular stimulation to improve ambulation after a cerebral vascular accident. *Phys Ther*, *59*(4), 423–426.

Fife, T. (August 1995). Horizontal canal benign positional vertigo. *ENG Rep*, 1–4.

Fischer, B., & Ramsperger, E. (1986). Human express saccades: effects of randomization and daily practice. *Exp Brain Res*, *64*, 569–578.

Fujino, A., Tokmasu, K., Okamoto, M., Naganuma, H., Hishino, I., Arai, M., et al. (1996). Vestibular training for acute unilateral vestibular disturbances: its efficacy in comparison with an anti-vertigo drug. *Acta Otolaryngol (Stockh) Suppl*, *524*, 21–26.

Gacek, R. R. (1991). Singular neurectomy update, II: A review of 102 cases. *Laryngoscope*, *101*, 855–862.

Gill-Body, K. M., Popat, R. A., Parker, S. W., & Krebs, D. E. (1997). Rehabilitation of balance function in patients with cerebellar dysfunction. *Phys Ther*, *77*(5), 534–551.

Gresty, M. A., Hess, K., & Leech, J. (1977). Disorders of the vestibulo-ocular reflex producing oscillopsia and mechanisms compensating for loss of labyrinthine function. *Brain*, *100*, 693–716.

Haupt, B. J., & Graves, E. (1982). Detailed diagnosis and surgical procedures for patients discharged from short stay hospitals. U.S. Dept. of Health and Human Services. DHHS Publication (PHS) 82-1274-1.

Hecker, H. C., Haug, C. O., & Herndon, J. W. (1974). Treatment of the vertiginous patient using Cawthorne's vestibular exercises. *Laryngoscope*, *84*, 2065–2072.

Herdman, S. J. (1994). Assessment and management of bilateral vestibular loss. In: S. J. Herdman (Ed.), *Vestibular rehabilitation* (pp. 316–330). Philadelphia: F.A. Davis.

Herdman, S. J. (1997). Advances in the treatment of vestibular disorders. *Phys Ther*, *77*(6), 602–617.

Herdman, S. J. (2001). Therapy: Rehabilitation. In: J. A Goebel (Ed.), *Practical management of the dizzy patient* (pp. 327–344). Philadelphia: Lippincott–Williams & Wilkins.

Herdman, S. J., & Tusa, R. J. (1996). Complications of the canalith repositioning procedure. *Arch Otolaryngol Head Neck Surg*, *122*, 281–286.

Herdman, S. J., & Tusa, R. J. (1999). *Benign paroxysmal positional vertigo*. Sechaumberg, Illinois: ICS Medical Corporation.

Herdman, S. J., Tusa, R. J., Zee, D. S., Proctor, L. R., & Mattox, D. E. (1993). Single treatment approaches to benign paroxysmal positional vertigo. *Arch Otolaryngol Head Neck Surg*, *119*, 450–454.

Hood, J. D. (1970). The clinical significance of vestibular rehabilitation. *Ann Otol Rhinol Laryngol*, *17*, 149–157.

Horak, F. B., Jones-Rycewicz, C., Black, F. O., & Shumway-Cook, A. (1992). Effects of vestibular rehabilitation on dizziness and imbalance. *Arch Otolaryngol Head Neck Surg*, *106*, 175–180.

Igarashi, M., Levy, J. K., O-Uchi, T., & Reschke, M. F. (1981). Further study of physical exercise and locomotor balance compensation after unilateral labyrinthectomy in squirrel monkeys. *Acta Otolaryngol*, *92*, 101–105.

Jacobson, G. P., & Newman, C. W. (1990). The development of the dizziness handicap inventory. *Arch Otolaryngol Head Neck Surg*, *116*, 424–427.

Karlberg, M. K., Hall, K., Quickert, N., Hinson, J. & Halmagyi, G. M. (2000). What inner ear diseases cause benign paroxysmal positional vertigo? *Acta Otolaryngol*, *120*, 380–385.

Kasai, T., & Zee, D. (1978). Eye–head coordination in labyrinthine-defective human beings. *Brain Res*, *144*, 123–141.

Lacour, M., Roll, J. P., & Appaix, M. (1976). Modifications and development of spinal reflexes in the alert baboon *(Papio papio)* following an unilateral vestibular neurectomy. *Brain Res*, *113*, 255–269.

Leigh, R. J., & Brandt, T. (1993). A re-evaluation of the vestibulo-ocular reflex: new ideas of its purpose, properties, neural substrate, and disorders. *Neurology*, *43*, 1288–1295.

Leigh, R. J., Sawyer, R. N., Grant, M. P., & Seidman, S. H. (1992). High-frequency vestibuloocular reflex as a diagnostic tool. *Ann New York Acad Sci*, *656*, 305–314.

Leigh, R. J., Sharpe, J. A., Ranalli, P. J., Thurston, S. E., & Hamid, M. A. (1987). Comparison of smooth pursuit and combined eye–head tracking in human subjects with deficient labyrinthine function. *Exp Brain Res*, *66*, 458–464.

Leigh, R. J., & Zee, D. S. (1991). *The neurology of eye movements* 2nd ed. Philadelphia: F.A. Davis.

Lempert, T., & Tiel-Wilck, K. (1996). A positional manuever for treatmentof horizontal-canal benign positional vertigo. *Laryngoscope*, *106*(4), 476–478..

Li, J. C. (1995). Mastoid oscillation: a critical factor for success in the canalith repositioning procedure. *Otolaryngol Head Neck Surg*, *112*, 670–675.

Lynn, S., Pool, A., Rose, D., Brey, R., & Suman, V. (1995). Randomized trial of the canalith repositioning procedure. *Otolaryngol Head Neck Surg*, *113*(6), 712–719.

McCabe, B. F. (1970). Labyrinthine exercises in the treatment of diseases characterized by vertigo: their physiologic basis and methodology. *Laryngoscope*, *80*, 1429–1433.

McKenzie, K. G. (1936). Intracranial division of the vestibular portion of the auditory nerve for Meniere's disease. *Can Med Assoc J*, *34*, 369–381.

Mathog, R. H., & Peppard, S. B. (1982). Exercise and recovery from vestibular injury. *Am J Otolaryngol*, *3*, 397–407.

Minor, L. B. (1999). Intratympanic gentamicin for control of vertigo in Meniere's disease: vestibular signs that specify completion of therapy. *Am J Otolaryngol*, *20*(2), 209–219.

Mira, E., Valli, S., Zucca, G., & Valli, P. (1996). Why do episodes of benign paroxysmal positioning vertigo recover spontaneously? *J Vestib Res Equilib Orient*, *6* (4s), S49.

Moffatt, D. A., & Ballagh, R. H. (1997). Meniere's disease. In: A. G. Kerr (Ed.), Scott-*Brown's otolaryngology*, pp. (3/19/1–3/19/50). 6th ed. Oxford: Butterworth-Heineman.

Murofushi, T., Halmagyi, G. M., & Yavor, R. A. (1997). Intratympanic gentamicin in Meniere's disease: Results of therapy. *Am J Otol*, *18*, 52–57.

Norre, M. E., & Beckers, A. (1987). Exercise treatment for paroxysmal positional vertigo: comparison of two types of exercise. *Arch Otol Rhinol Laryngol*, *244*, 291–294.

Norre, M. E., & Beckers, A. (1988). Comparative study of two types of exercise treatment for paroxysmal positioning vertigo. *Advances in Oto-Rhino-Laryngology*, *42*, 287–289.

Norre, M. E., & DeWeert, W. (1980). Treatment of vertigo based on habituation: technique and results for habituation training. *J Laryngol Otol*, *94*, 971–977.

Odkvist, L. M., Bergenius, J., & Miller, C. (1997). When and how to use gentamicin in the treatment of Menieres' disease. *Acta Otolaryngol (Stockh) Suppl*, *526*, 54–57.

Parnes, L. S., & McClure, J. A. (1990). Posterior semicircular canal occlusion for intractable benign positional vertigo. *Ann Otol Rhinol Laryngol*, *99* (5 pt 1), 330–333.

Parnes, L. S., & Price-Jones, R. G. (1993). Particle repositioning maneuver for benign paroxysmal positional vertigo. *Ann Otol Rhinol Laryngol*, *102* (5), 325–331.

Parnes, L. S., & Robichaud, J. (1997). Further observations during the particle repositioning maneuver for benign paroxysmal positional vertigo. *Otolaryngol Head Neck Surg*, *116* (2), 238–243.

Parry, R. H. (1904). A case of tinnitus and vertigo treated by division of the auditory nerve. *J Laryngol Rhinol Otol*, *91*, 402–406.

Pfaltz, C. R. (1983). Vestibular compensation. *Acta Otolaryngol*, *95*, 402–406.

Pfaltz, C. R., & Kamath, R. (1971). The problem of central compensation of peripheral vestibular disorders. *Acta Otolaryngol*, *71*, 266–272.

Portman, G. (1927). The saccus endolymphaticus and an operation for draining the same for the relief of vertigo. *J Laryngol Otol*, *42*, 809.

Radtke, A., Neuhauser, H., von Brevern, M., & Lempert, T. (1999). A modified Epley's procedure for self-treatment of benign paroxysmal positional vertigo. *Neurology*, *53*, 1358–1360.

Sawyer, R. M., Thurston, S. E., Becker, K. R., Ackley, C. V., Seidman, S. H., & Leigh, J. R. (1994). The cervico-ocular reflex of normal human subjects in response to transient and sinusoidal trunk rotations. *J Vestib Res*, *4* (3), 245–249.

Schuknecht, H. F. (1957). Ablation therapy in the management of Meniere's disease. *Acta Otolaryngol Suppl (Stockh)*, *132*, 1–42.

Schuknecht, H. F. (1969). Cupulolithiasis. *Arch Otolaryngol Head Neck Surg*, *90*, 765–778.

Semont, A., Freyss, G., & Vitte, E. (1988). Curing the BPPV with a liberatory maneuver. *Ann Otol Rhinol Laryngol*, *42*, 290–293.

Serafini, G., Palmieri, A. M. R., & Simoncelli, C. (1996). Benign paroxysmal positional vertigo of posterior semicircular canal: results in 160 cases treated with Semont's maneuver. *Ann Otol Rhinol Laryngol*, *105*, 770–774.

Shea, J. J. (1989). Perfusion of the inner ear with streptomycin. *Am J Otol*, *102*, 150–155.

Shepard, N. T., & Telian, S. A. (1995). Programmatic vestibular rehabilitation. *Otolaryngol Head Neck Surg*, *112* (1), 173–182.

Shepard, N. T., & Telian, S. A. (1996). *Practical management of the balance disorder patient*. San Diego: Singular Publishing Group.

Shepard, N. T., Telian, S. A., & Smith-Wheelock, M. (1990). Habituation and balance retraining therapy: a retrospective review. *Neurol Clin North Am*, *8* (2), 459–475.

Shepard, N. T., Telian, S. A., & Smith-Wheelock, M. (1993). Vestibular and balance rehabilitation therapy. *Ann Otol Rhinol Laryngol*, *102*, 198–205.

Silverstein, H., Rosenberg, S., Arruda, J., & Isaacson, J. E. (1997). Surgical ablation of the vestibular system in the treatment of Meniere's disease. *Otolaryngol Clin North Am*, *30* (6), 1075–1095.

Silverstein, H., Smouha, E., & Jones, E. (1989). Natural history vs. surgery for Meniere's disease. *Arch Otolaryngol*, *107*, 271–277.

Sloane, P. D., Dallara, J., Roach, C., Bailey, K. E., Mitchell, M., & McNutt, R. (1994). Management of dizziness in primary care. *J Am Board Fam Pract*, *7*, 1–8.

Smith, P. F., Darlington, C. L., & Curthoys, I. S. (1986). The effect of visual deprivation on vestibular compensation in the guinea pig. *Brain Res*, *364*, 195–198.

Steddin, S., & Brandt, T. (1996). Horizontal canal benign paroxysmal positioning vertigo (h-bppv): Transitioning of canalithiasis to cupulothiasis. *Ann Neurol, 40*, 918–922.

Steenerson, R., & Cronin, G. (1996). Comparison of the canalith repositioning procedure and vestibular habituation training in forty patients with benign paroxysmal positional vertigo. *Otolaryngol Head Neck Surg, 114*(1), 61–64.

Stockwell, C. (1996, May). Tutorial on the three forms of benign positional vertigo (BPV). Schaumberg, Illinois: ICS Medical, 1–5.

Szturm, T., Ireland, D. J., & Lessing-Turner, M. (1994). Comparison of different exercise programs in the rehabilitation of patients with chronic peripheral vestibular dysfunction. *J Vestib Res, 4*(6), 461–479.

Thomsen, J., Bretlau, P., Tos, M., & Johnson, N. J. (1981). Placebo effect for surgery for Meniere's disease. *Arch Otolaryngol, 107*, 271–277.

Tideiksaar, R. (1989). Medical causes of falling. In: R. Tideiksaar, R., (Ed.), *Falling in old age: Its prevention and treatment* (pp. 21–47). New York: Springer.

Tinetti, M. E., & Williams, C. S. (1997). Falls, injuries due to falls, and risk of admission to a nursing home. *N Engl J Med, 337*(18), 1279–1284.

Toupet, M., & Semont, A. (1985). La physiotherapie du vertige paroxystique benin. In: R. Hausler (Ed.), *Les Vertiges d'origine peripherique et centrale* (pp. 21–27). Paris: Ibsen.

Trine, M. B., Lynn, S. G., Facer, G. W., & Kasperbauer, J. L. (1995). Intratympanic gentamicin treatment: preliminary results in two patients with Meniere's disease. *J Am Acad Audiol, 6*, 264–270.

van Deelen, G. W., & Huizing, E. H. (1986). Use of a diuretic (Dyazide) in the treatment of Meniere's disease. *Otorhinolaryngology, 48*, 287–292.

Webster's New World Dictionary. (1976). D. B. Guralnik (Ed.). Cleveland: William Collins & World Publishing.

Yamane, H., Imoto, T., Nakai, Y., Igarashi, M., & Rask-Anderson, H. (1984). Otoconia degradation. *Acta Otolaryngol Suppl, 406*, 263–270.

Yardley, L., Burgneay, J., Anderson, G., Owen, N., Nazareth, J., & Luxon, L. (1998). Feasibility and effectiveness of providing vestibular rehabilitation for dizzy patients in the community. *Clin Otolaryngol, 23*, 442–448.

Zee, D. (1985). Perspectives on the pharmacotherapy of vertigo. *Arch Otolaryngol, 111*, 609–612.

7

Staffing Needs of the Balance Clinic

Preparing to offer comprehensive evaluations and treatments for patients with vestibular disorders requires research, planning, and sufficient capital. These factors pale when compared with the amount of training and experience required to operate a balance clinic competently. The balance and vestibular system is complex, and one cannot proclaim oneself a "vestibular specialist" without substantial training additional to that required to obtain a degree or licensure.

Dizziness and dysequilibrium can occur from disruptions in one or more of the sensory systems responsible for balance, from the inaccurate integration of those signals, or from insufficient motor control. The cause may be related to a reaction with medication, or it may be the result of a psychiatric condition. No single medical or allied health specialty can provide an "expert opinion" for all possible causes of dizziness. No formal training programs offer degrees as a "vestibular specialist." The comprehensive evaluation and treatment of the dizzy patient require a multidisciplinary team approach, which minimally consists of a medical director (typically otolaryngology or neurology), audiology, and physical therapy. Occupational therapists, physiatrists, psychologists, and nurses also participate as part of the "balance clinic" team.

The team approach for staffing a balance clinic has numerous advantages. The patient receives the benefit of seeing several specialists, at one site, on one day (see Appendix D for a sample patient flow sheet). Typically, the entry point at a balance clinic will involve some type of screening(s) to determine what specialists and what examinations may be most helpful to address the patient's complaints. This screening examination can be performed by any member of the team who has been trained and is experienced in taking a case history and performing screening examinations (see Chapter 3). The team members have the benefit of interacting with other team members to discuss their findings and how these findings may relate to a final diagnosis. The payers (a third party or the patient) benefit from cost savings related to reduced duplication of services, faster diagnosis, and treatment leading to less time lost from work and improved likelihood of effective treatment.

"Vestibular Specialists"

None of the above specialties should consider themselves as "vestibular specialists" simply by virtue of obtaining their degree and licensure. Currently no specific requirements exist that dictate which specialty will be involved in the care of the dizzy patient, nor are there specific guidelines as to what role each specialty should play. Historically, some professionals in each and all the above-listed specialties have focused their practice on vestibular disorders and have received training over and above that required to obtain the designated degree and licensure.

Inevitably, some controversy remains over "who should be doing what," and occasionally the issue of "turf-battles" has arisen. The concept of multispecialty balance clinics is relatively new, and the turf battle issue is unsettled. Rather than offer any opinion or argument as to what is considered appropriate practice for each of the listed specialties, a review of applicable scope of practice and position statements is included. Readers may then establish their own opinion and contribute to the discussion of "who should be doing what."

Scope of Practice

Scope of Practice Evolution

It is important to recognize that, as technologies develop and new diagnostic and treatment modalities become part of clinical practice, the scope of practice guidelines change as well. Givens (1994) lists four aspects involved in the natural evolution of a profession's scope of practice:

1. Legal limitations must be established which define appropriate practice within the profession. It is acknowledged that legal statutes typically lag behind clinical practice in an evolving, dynamic profession.
2. Practitioners must constantly monitor changes and developments in knowledge, technology and health care delivery. Changes in practice should be reflected in changes in Scope of Practice statements, with consumer protection of utmost importance.
3. Professional training programs must change as the standard of clinical practice changes. Both practicing professionals and students must keep current with the latest practice techniques.
4. Statutes and regulations must be revised periodically to reflect the changes in the profession. Unlike scope of practice statements within a profession, changes in statutes and regulation are often affected by politics. Resistance to changes expanding legal definitions of scope of practice may be offered from other professions concerned with protecting their "turf."

Givens (1994) suggests that there is a natural tug of war between allowing scope of practice statements to promote growth within a profession and protecting consumers from legally allowing untrained practitioners from engaging in activities they may not be adequately trained to perform.

Role of Otolaryngology

The role of the otolaryngologist typically includes acting as medical director of the clinic. Because a significant number of patients complaining of dizziness are ultimately found to have vestibular dysfunction, an otolaryngologist has unique training in ear disease and in the medical/surgical treatment of otologic disorders known to cause dizziness. Otolaryngologists are board certified by the American Academy of Otolaryngology–Head and Neck Surgery (AAO-HNS). The scope of practice set forth by the AAO-HNS does not set specific guidelines regarding management of vestibular dysfunction, but there are several policy statements (listed herein) related to certain aspects of vestibular testing and treatment.

Policy Statement 1360: The Scope of Otoloaryngology–Head and Neck Surgery

The American Academy of Otolaryngology–Head and Neck surgery agrees with the policy of the American Medical Association that surgeons should be allowed to do all procedures for which they are qualified by training and experience. Otolaryngologists–head and neck surgeons are, by training, regional physicians and surgeons of the head and neck. Included within the field are those measures associated with the restoration or improvement of form and function of structures of the head and neck. This may require harvesting of tissues from other anatomical areas. Surgery performed in an anatomical area outside of the head and neck not primarily relating to the treatment of conditions involving the head and neck is considered to be outside the scope of otolaryngology–head and neck surgery.

Adopted 5/14/84, revised 9/16/95, reaffirmed 3/1/98

Policy Statement 1160: Dynamic Posturography and Vestibular Testing

The American Academy of Otolaryngology–Head and Neck Surgery recognizes that the following tests or treatments are medically appropriate in the evaluation or treatment of persons with suspected vestibular disorders:

1. Harmonic acceleration testing
2. Vestibular rehabilitation therapy
3. Dynamic platform posturography, under the circumstances detailed in the Technology Assessment prepared by the Academy Task Force on Posturography.

Adopted 7/20/90, reaffirmed 4/13/95, revised 9/21/98.

Policy Statement 1460: Vestibular Rehabilitation/Balance Retraining Therapy

Vestibular rehabilitation, or balance retraining therapy (BRT), is a scientifically based and clinically valid therapeutic modality for the treatment of persistent dizziness and postural instability due to incomplete compensation after peripheral vestibular or central nervous system injury. Balance retraining therapy is also a significant benefit for fall prevention in the elderly after suffering from multiple sensory and motor impairment.

Adopted 6/28/97, reaffirmed 3/1/98

Reprinted with permission from the Academy of Otolaryngology–Head and Neck Surgery Bulletin, *October 1998. Vol. 17, 10*.

The Academy of Otolaryngology–Head and Neck Surgery also periodically issues a "Clinical Indicators" statement that provides guidelines for the use of particular procedures. The AAO-HNS warns, "in no way do they represent a standard of care. The applicability of an indicator for a procedure, and/or of the process or outcome criteria, must be determined by the responsible physician in light of all the circumstances presented by the individual patient. Adherence to these guidelines will not ensure successful treatment in every situation." The AAO-HNS "emphasizes that these clinical indicators should not be deemed inclusive of all proper treatment decisions or methods of care, nor exclusive of other treatment decisions or methods of care reasonably directed to obtaining the same results" (AOO-HNS Bulletin, 2000).

The Clinical Indicators for Canalith Repositioning follow:

Canalith Repositioning

(Otolith Repositioning; Epley Maneuver; Semont Maneuver)

Procedure	CPT	FUD	Additional Information
Therapeutic procedure, one or more areas, each 15 minutes; neuromuscular reeducation of balance, coordination, or kinesthetic sense	97112	XXX	Assistant Surgeon - None Supply Charge - L0120 Cervical Collar Anesthesia Codes - None
Manual therapy techniques; One or more regions; each 15 minutes	97140	XXX	
Therapeutic activities, direct patient contact by the provider (one on one) dynamic activities to improve functional performance each 15 minutes	97530	XXX	

Indications

1.   History
     a)   Description of vertigo.
     b)   Functional impairment due to vertigo.
     c)   History of head trauma.

    d)   History of upper respiratory infection.
    e)   No evidence of neck or back disorders that might contraindicate this maneuver.

2.   Physical Examination
    a)   Neurotologic examination
        *Hallpike maneuver.
        *Spontaneous or gaze nystagmus.
        *Cranial nerve testing
    b)   Cerebellar examination
    c)   Carotid artery auscultation

3.   Tests (optional)
    a)   Audiometry
    b)   Electronystagmography (ENG)

Outcome Review

1.   First Month
        Presence or absence of positional vertigo.
2.   Beyond One Month
        Presence of absence of positional vertigo.
        Resumption of normal life style.
        Consideration for further evaluation if symptoms persist.

Therapeutic

Patient Information

Benign positional vertigo is one of the most common causes of dizziness seen by the otolaryngologist. This inner ear problem is caused by crystals floating in the fluid of the inner ear. On position change, these crystals stimulate part of the inner ear and produce short periods of dizziness. Causes for the crystals to break away are: head injuries, decreased blood to the inner ear, degenerative diseases, and viral infections of the inner ear or are unknown. This process usually takes from one to 12 months to occur. In time, these crystals will settle, and the symptoms will go away.

The crystals can be repositioned to shorten the time it takes for positional vertigo to resolve. This repositioning is called the Epley or Semont maneuver. This is a simple in-office therapy that takes about 30 minutes. The patient is placed in several different positions during the maneuver which usually causes temporary dizziness. Patients may wear a neck collar overnight to help keep the head and neck in position. Many patients have improvement with this treatment or repeated treatments. Reprinted from AOO-HNS Bulletin, 2000.

The editorial in Box 7–1 highlights the fact that most patients with vestibular disorders require management techniques that are not emphasized in typical otolaryngology residencies. Since this editorial was written in 1992, the AAO-HNS has taken steps to increase the exposure to vestibular management in its training programs.

Box 7–1

Editorial_____

Training the Balance Specialist

In this decade of highly specialized medicine, post-residency training is often required to achieve skills for managing certain highly technical medical and surgical problems. Neurotology, with its unique blend of medical neurology and surgical procedures, exemplifies this challenge. Unfortunately, many existing fellowship training programs for neurotology emphasize surgical expertise at the expense of diagnostic and therapeutic skills required for the treatment of the entire spectrum of balance disorders.

In our vestibular laboratory at Washington University School of Medicine, we examine, test, and treat over 500 patients a year. Of these, fewer than 5% ever require an operation. This low incidence of surgical cases among all patients referred for dizziness already has been noted in the literature. In the majority of cases, a careful evaluation based on history, physical findings, and laboratory test results, followed by a thoughtful explanation of the condition and an ongoing therapeutic program, is required for optimal benefit. With this in mind, any specialist who is trained exclusively in surgery often finds both himself and his patients frustrated. On the other hand, if the balance expert understands the multisensory nature of balance and posture control and, in addition, masters all aspects of therapy (pharmacotherapy, conditioning programs, formal rehabilitation, lifestyle alterations, and surgery), then most patients will benefit greatly from their interaction.

The time has come to reconsider and broaden the goals of post-residency training in neurotology. As a general rule, the graduate fellow from any program should understand all available diagnostic tools (ENG, rotary chair, posturography, audiologic, and radiographic studies) and treatment options both medical and surgical. More critical than any operation it is the decision-making process to select appropriate candidates for surgery. Most important, for the larger group of patients who are not candidates for surgery, the graduating neurologist must be able to offer a reasonable explanation of the problem and a workable therapeutic plan with the optimal combination of physical rehabilitation, lifestyle alteration, and drug therapy. Only in this fashion will the balance specialist be able to help these challenging patients.

Joel A. Goebel, M.D.

Mattox, D. E. (1980). Medical management of vertigo. *Ear Nose Throat J, 59*(10):5–13.

Brandt, T., Daroff, R. B. (1980). Physical therapy for benign paroxysmal positional vertigo. *Arch Otolaryngol, 1066*, 484-485.

Smyth, G. D. L., Hassard, T. H., Kerr, A. G. (1981). The surgical treatment of vertigo. Essentials of patient selection and long-term results. *Am J Otol*, 22:179– 187.

Reprinted with permission from The American Journal of Otology, 1992.

Role of Neurology

Although epidemiologic studies indicate that the minority of dizzy patients are found to have neurologic disorders (Kroenke, Hoffman, & Einstadter, 2000; Kroenke et al., 1992; Lawson, Fitzgerald, Birchall, Aldren, & Kenny, 1999), primary care doctors have indicated that they are more likely to make a specialty referral when a neurologic (as opposed to an otologic) cause is suspected (Sloane, Hartman, & Mitchell, 1994). Neurologists may be board certified through the American Academy of Neurology, which has issued a technical report outlining the academies position on the use of electronystagmography. The "executive summary" of this report follows:

> Electronystagmography, based upon class III evidence (i.e., evidence provided by expert opinion, nonrandomized historical controls, or case reports of one or more), with a type C strength of recommendation, is considered an established test of vestibulo-ocular function that is both safe and effective. Because of the particular importance of test administration and test interpretation, it is recommended that electronystagmography be performed by persons who have the requisite skills, ability, knowledge and experience. Under these conditions, can provide clinically useful information for the diagnosis of the vestibular system abnormalities including disorders that affect the peripheral or central vestibular system. Electronystagmography testing is a specialized tool that should be reserved for the assessment of patients with vertigo, dizziness, or dysequilibrium who are suspected of suffering from a vestibular system abnormality." (Neurology, 1996)

Role of Audiology

The role of the audiologist in the diagnostic workup of the dizzy patient is well established, although some preeminent audiologists have made the argument that audiologists should focus on the diagnosis and treatment of hearing (or communication) disorders only. It has been argued that audiologists can only serve in a subordinate role and that involvement in the management of vestibular patients may undermine the ability of the audiologist to be an autonomous professional (Turner, 1992). Audiologists are well established as the provider of choice for audiometric assessment, which is an integral aspect of a comprehensive vestibular evaluation. Audiologists also traditionally perform electronystagmography (ENG) and other vestibular tests. A recent survey of audiologists (Martin, Champlin, & Chambers, 1998) reports that 47% of responding audiologists are performing ENG examinations. This represents a significant increase from 34% performing ENG examinations in 1985. Sixty-eight percent of responding audiologists believed that an audiologist should perform the ENG examination, whereas 18% felt that a technician or support personnel should perform the examination. Only 5% thought audiologists should have no role in the administration or interpretation of ENG examinations, whereas 80% believed that audiologists should both perform and interpret ENG examinations.

The role of the audiologist in the treatment of patients with vestibular dysfunction is less well established and has been the subject of a recent, lengthy position statement issued by the American Speech Language and Hearing Association (ASHA). An additional confounding variable is the fact that audiologists have two governing bodies: ASHA and the American Academy of Audiology (AAA). Both these organizations have issued scope of practice statements, which take slightly different positions on the role of audiologists in the treatment of vestibular disorders.

Role of Audiologists in Vestibular and Balance Rehabilitation: Position Statement, Guidelines, and Technical Report

---

ASHA Ad Hoc Committee on Vestibular Rehabilitation

This position statement is an official policy of the American Speech-Language-Hearing Association (ASHA). It was developed by the Ad Hoc Committee on Vestibular Rehabilitation and adopted by the ASHA Legislative Council (LC-A/HS 1-99) in January 1999, Members of the committee include Nancy P. Garrus; Eric B. Hecker; Kenneth G. Henry; Susan Herdman, Ph.D., PT, consultant; Neil T. Shepard, chair; Charles W. Stockwell; and Maureen E. Thompson, ex officio. Richard Nodar, vice president for professional practices in audiology, served as monitoring vice president.

Position Statement

It is the position of the American Speech-Language-Hearing Association (ASHA) that the following two areas of practice are within the scope of practice of audiologists who possess the general and specific knowledge and skills for these specific areas outlined in the ASHA Guidelines on the Role of Audiologists in Vestibular and Balance Rehabilitation:

1. Canalith repositioning procedures (CRP), which consists of various methods of specific movements of the head and body designs to reposition otoconia and/or other material from abnormal location in one of the semicircular canals back into the vestibule region.
2. Consultation to and/or serving as a member of a multidisciplinary team managing patients with balance disorders and/or dizziness.

Reference this material as: American Speech-Language-Hearing Association. (1999, March). Role of audiologists in vestibular and balance rehabilitation; Position statement, guidelines, and technical report. *Asha*, 41 (Suppl. 19), 13–22.

Index terms: benign paroxysmal positioning vertigo (BBPV), canalith repositioning procedure, disequilibrium, electronystagmography, vestibular and balance rehabilitation

ASHA maintains that professionals must be specifically trained as outlined in the ASHA Guidelines on the Role of Audiologists in Vestibular and Balance Rehabilitation Programs.

Performance of vestibular and balance rehabilitation therapy (VBRT) by lesser-trained individuals could lead to suboptimal results, prolongation of therapy, and possible exacerbation of other concomitant medical conditions.

This position statement recognizes further that the area of VBRT is changing rapidly and there is no intention to preclude future VBRT techniques being included in the scope of practice for audiology.

Guidelines

These guidelines are an official statement of the American Speech-language-Hearing Association (ASHA). They provide guidance on the role of audiologists in vestibular and balance rehabilitation but are not official standards of the Association. These guidelines were adopted by the ASHA Executive Board (EB 64–98) in November 1998. These guidelines, which were developed from current literature and a course, Vestibular Rehabilitation: A Competency-Based Course, hosted by the Division of Physical Therapy, University of Miami School of Medicine, were recognized as being applicable to the profession of audiology. Members of the committee include Nancy P. Garrus; Eric B. Hecker; Kenneth G. Henry; Susan Herdman, Ph.D., PT, consultant; Neil T. Shepard, chair; Charles Stockwell, and Maureen Thompson, ex officio, Richard Nodar, vice president for professional practices in audiology, served as monitoring vice president.

Introduction

These guidelines were developed from current literature and from a course offered to physical and occupational therapies, Vestibular Rehabilitation: A Competency-Based Course, sponsored by the University of Miami School of Medicine, Division of Physical Therapy and held March 12–14, 1998, in Miami, FL. The course director, Susan J. Herdman, Ph.D., PT, served as a consultant to this committee. The course consisted of three days of lecture, laboratory sessions, and self-study sessions. In order to successfully complete the course, participants were expected to demonstrate the following assessment skills: oculomotor examination, with emphasis on the identification of nystagmus and canal involvement; balance and gait; fall risk; and functional assessments. Participants were also expected to demonstrate appropriate treatment procedures for benign paroxysmal positional vertigo (BBPV) affecting posterior, anterior, and horizontal canals for both cupulolithiasis and canalithiasis, for unilateral and bilateral peripheral vestibular disorders, and for central vestibular disorders, including traumatic brain injury and stroke. Members of the ASHA Ad Hoc Committee and Vestibular Rehabilitation recognized that these competencies were applicable to the profession of audiology.

Background

Historically, audiologists have been involved in the assessment of patients with balance disorders and/or dizziness and imbalance utilizing procedures such as electronystagmography (ENG), rotational tests, oculomotor tests, and dynamic posturography. These assessment procedures have expanded the role and responsibilities of the Audiologist to include participation on the rehabilitation team for patients identified with balance system dysfunction. Vestibular and balance rehabilitation therapy (VBRT) encompasses a formulation of exercise activities, preferably customized to the needs of the patient, designed to promote the system's natural central compensation process that reduces and, in some cases, eliminates symptoms for the patient with chronic balance disorders and/or dizziness. Audiologists may be involved in the administration of canalith repositioning procedures (CRP), a portion of a full VBRT program, and as consultants on multidisciplinary teams providing overall management to these patients.

These guidelines are designed to serve as a model for audiologists who are interested in (a) performing canalith repositioning maneuvers, and (b) serving as consultants to or members of multidisciplinary teams managing the patient with balance disorders and/or dizziness. The guidelines specify the knowledge and skills required to perform these tasks and the manner in which these skills may by acquired.

Education and Training

The education and practical experience for the broader area of full vestibular rehabilitation (i.e., providing full clinical assessment of patients and developing rehabilitation activities including but not limited to CRP, gait and balance, adaptation and habituation exercise, as discussed in ASHA's Technical Report on Vestibular & Balance Rehabilitation Programs) is not typically available in audiology educational training programs or in typical postgraduate audiology courses. This type of extensive education involves graduate level work in physical and/or occupational therapy or other disciplines in addition to postgraduate course work in these other disciplines.

At this time, academic programs in audiology do offer a limited education and practical experience in balance system assessment and canalith repositioning techniques. A limited portion of the required knowledge and skills may be obtained from graduate level studies in the anatomy and physiology of the balance system. Therefore, audiologists typically obtain most knowledge and skills through postgraduate continuing education courses in audiology and other disciplines (e.g., physical or occupational therapy, neurology).

The Certificate of Clinical Competence in Audiology (CCC-A) from ASHA ensures that audiologists have met the entry level education, knowledge, and experience requirements established by the Association for providing clinical services in the profession of audiology. In order to perform the clinical procedures discussed in this document, audiologists typically possess knowledge and skills beyond those obtained through "entry level" education. All audiologists who are interested in performing CRP and serving as consultants to and/or members of multidisciplinary teams managing patients with balance disorders and/or dizziness should ensure that they have acquired the general and specific knowledge and skills outlined below.

The ASHA Code of Ethics (ASHA, 1994) states:

Individuals shall honor their responsibility to achieve and maintain high standards of professional competence. (Principle of Ethics II)

The Code of Ethics also states:

Individuals shall engage only in those aspects of their profession that are within the scope of their competence, considering their level of education, training, and experience. (Principle of Ethics II, Rule B)

The extent to which audiologists may be involved in the CRP portion of vestibular and balance rehabilitation programs is dependent on their current knowledge and skill level, privileges granted within a specific job setting, state licensure requirements, and the type of vestibular/balance assessment and rehabilitation management program available.

Other professionals in related fields also may be involved with the rehabilitation of patients with balance disorders and/or dizziness and it is not ASHA's intent to exclude or influence their participation.

Knowledge and Skills

Outlined below are the general and specific objectives and skills required by audiologists who intend to develop and/or administer CRP and/or intend to serve as consultants on multidisciplinary teams managing patients who have balance disorders and/or dizziness.

General Knowledge and Skills

A. Objective: Knowledge of the anatomy and physiology of the subsystems necessary for balance maintenance.

Knowledge/skills needed: General knowledge of the anatomy and physiology of the peripheral and central vestibular, visual and somatosensory/proprioceptive system and their relative interaction.

B. Objective: Knowledge of the pathophysiology of the balance system and the subjective and somatic complaints that lead to imbalance and/or dizziness.

Knowledge/skills needed: Knowledge of various pathological processes that can affect the sensory and motor subsystems responsible for normal balance and equilibrium.

C. Objective: Understanding of the general management techniques used for the treatment of vestibular and balance disorders.

Knowledge/skills needed: In addition to the requisite skills and knowledge necessary for the management of CRP, the audiologist should be familiar with other management techniques and when these might be used to include other activities in the area of vestibular and balance rehabilitation, medical, surgical or dietary strategies for the patient with a balance disorder and/or dizziness.

D. Objective: Ability to determine appropriate candidacy for vestibular and balance rehabilitation.

Knowledge/skills needed: The audiologist should possess the ability to determine potential candidacy for basic rehabilitation based on the patient's presenting history and symptoms supplemented by presenting signs (e.g., nystagmus), laboratory tests, functional assessment and rule out alternative methods of treatment or contraindication to vestibular rehabilitation by the patient's managing physician.

Specific Knowledge/Skills – Assessment

A. Objective: Interpretation and integration of diagnostic vestibular tests and other laboratory data for diagnostic and functional assessment.

Knowledge/skills needed: Possess the ability to interpret and integrate various laboratory studies for the purposes of diagnostic evaluation as well as to establish a baseline for outcome measures to assess the efficacy of rehabilitation and other management techniques. These tests may include but are not limited to: ENG including, extensive oculomotor evaluation; rotational chair; head and body rotation; postural control assessment; audiological evaluation; electrocochleography; auditory brainstem evoked potentials.

B. Objective: Possess the ability to perform and interpret a variety of direct clinical evaluations designed for diagnostic assessment of the patient with disorders of the balance system.

Knowledge/skills needed: Skill with techniques for direct clinical examinations for diagnostic and rehabilitative assessments. These may include but not limited to:

- Oculomotor to examinations with and without visual fixation (ocular alignment; spontaneous and gaze-holding nystagmus;

ocular range of motion; vergence; pursuit and saccade eye movements; vestibulo-ocular reflex (VOR) cancellation; VOR to slow head rotation; VOR to head thrusts; head-shaking nystagmus; pressure-induced nystagmus; hyperventilation-induced nystagmus; dynamic visual acuity testing; vertebral artery compression test; Dix-Hallpike); and
- Balance and gait evaluation (Romberg; tandem Romberg; modified clinical test for sensory interaction and balance (CTSIB); Fukuda stepping test; gait analysis; tandem walk).

C. Objective: Ability to determine presence of posterior canal BPPV or anterior and horizontal canal variants causing symptoms of dizziness.

Knowledge/skills needed: Knowledge of and ability to perform a clinical assessment of maneuvers that provoke symptoms associated with posterior canal BPPV or its anterior and horizontal variants. The tools may include but not be limited to:

- Dix-Hallpikc maneuver to assess posterior and anterior canal BPPV;
- Side-lying test for BPPV; and
- Roll test for horizontal canal BPPV.

D. Objective: Assess effects of ongoing medical conditions that might influence the CRP.

Knowledge/skills needed: Ability to assess the impact of general medical conditions and knowledge of specific conditions that might compromise or contraindicate a CRP.

Specific Knowledge/Skills – Treatment

A. Objective: Perform, when indicated by diagnosis and direct examination, canalith repositioning procedures for canalithiasis or cupulolithiasis of the posterior, anterior or horizontal semicircular canals.

Knowledge/skills needed: Knowledge of the theory, rationale and procedures necessary to successfully distinguish between posterior, anterior and horizontal canal BPPV and between canalithiasis and cupulolithiasis; and skill to administer a canalith repositioning procedure on patients with BPPV of posterior, anterior or horizontal canal origin.

Precautions

Patients: CRP may result in patient discomfort or adverse reactions. It is the responsibility of the audiologist who conducts and supervises a CRP to develop specific protocols in conjuction with appropriate medical personnel to ensure patient safety and comfort. These protocols may include, but not be limited to:

1. Assurances that balance system assessments as well as vestibular and balance rehabilitation techniques are performed in a safe and comfortable environment.
2. Identification of personnel responsible for the administration and/or interpretation of balance system assessments as well as vestibular and balance rehabilitation programs.
3. Identification of appropriate medical personnel to contact in the event that emergency medical assistance is needed.
4. Provision of informed consent as required by the facility and/or regulatory bodies.
5. Documentation of patient conditions before, during, and following test administration and/or CRP.

Audiologist: It is recommended that audiologists adhere to the Universal Precautions outlined in the Center for Disease Control Morbidity and Mortality Weekly report (June 24, 1988, *Perspectives in Disease Prevention and Health Promotion*, 37 (24), 377–388.

Audiologists also must understand the potential for professional liability for any procedure they conduct or supervise. Institutional and/or regulatory bodies, such as state licensure boards, should be informed that CRP is within the scope of practice for audiology. Audiologists should ensure, where applicable, that no limitations have been imposed on their scope of practice that would restrict the coverage of these procedures under their professional liability policy.

The scope of practice statement of the ASHA provides a broad interpretation of their position of audiology's involvement in managing patients with vestibular dysfunction. A more comprehensive opinion is offered in the position statement on "The role of audiologists in vestibular rehabilitation: position statement, guidelines, and technical report." Listed are the entire position statement and applicable excerpts from ASHA's Scope of Practice in

Balance System Assessment

Ad Hoc Committee on Advances in Clinical Practice
American Speech-Language-Hearing Association

This policy statement was prepared by the American Speech-Language-Hearing Association (ASHA) Ad Hoc Committee on Advances in Clinical Practice: Donald E. Morgan, chair; Carol M. Frattali, ex officio; Zilpha T. Bosone; David G. Cyr; Deborah Hayes; Krysztof Izdebski; Paul Kileny; Neil T.

Shepard; Barbara C. Sonies; Jaclyn B. Spitzer; and Frank B. Wilson, Diane L. Eger, 1991–1993 vice president for professional practices, and Teris K. Schery, 1988–1990 vice president for clinical affairs, served as monitoring vice presidents. The contributions of the Executive Board, and select and wide-spread peer reviewers are gratefully acknowledged. The Legislative Council approved the document as official policy of the Association at its November 1991 meeting (LC 51A-91).

I. Introduction

Speech-language pathology and audiology are dynamic and expanding professions with constantly developing technological and clinical advances. Before conducting procedures involving such advances, practitioners must have acquired the knowledge, skills, education, and experience necessary to perform them competently. This policy statement is one of seven documents developed by the Ad Hoc Committee on Advances in Clinical Practice. Each statement expresses the position of the American Speech-Language-Hearing Association (ASHA) concerning specific clinical procedures within the scope of practice of speech-language pathology or audiology, most of which have developed within the last few years. Each statement further provides guidelines for practitioners performing these procedures.

The documents include Position Statements and Guidelines for Balance System Assessment, Electrical Stimulation for Cochlear Implant Selection and Rehabilitation, Evaluation and Treatment for Tracheoesophageal Fistulization/Puncture, External Auditory Canal Examination and Cerumen Management, Instrumental Diagnostic Procedures for Swallowing, Neurophysiologic: Intraoperative Monitoring, Vocal Tract Visualization and Imaging

The guidelines consider the knowledge and skills normally associated with required competencies, the clinical settings recommended for the procedure, and the appropriate involvement of personnel from other disciplines.

Clinical certification by ASHA ensures that practitioners have met the education, knowledge, and experience requirements established by the Association for providing basic clinical services in the professions of speech-language pathology or audiology. Certification in the appropriate profession is necessary, but not sufficient to perform the specific clinical procedure(s) discussed in this statement. The procedure(s) addressed in this document requires the practitioner to obtain education and training beyond that necessary for ASHA certification. Practitioners are bound by the ASHA Code of Ethics to maintain high standards of professional competence. Therefore, practitioners should engage only in those aspects of the professions that are within the scope of their level of education, training, and experience.

In promulgating this policy statement, there is no intention to imply that the practitioner holding ASHA Certification is prepared to conduct the procedure(s); nor is it incumbent on any certified professional to provide the procedure(s) merely because the practitioner holds certification.

The following document is intended as guidelines for the practitioner to ensure the quality of care, welfare, safety, and comfort of those served by our professions.

II. Background

Audiologists, historically, have been involved in the assessment of patients with dizziness and imbalance. Recent surveys have indicated that a significant number of audiologists are continuing this trend (Martin & Morris, 1989). The improvement and expansion of balance function assessment (e.g., computerized electronystagmography (ENG)/ocular motor tests, rotational tests of the vestibular-ocular reflex (VOR), and dynamic posturography) have expanded the role and responsibilities of audiologists involved in this area of assessment. In addition, the emergence of state-of-the-art assessment procedures has led to a relatively new area of interest dealing with (re)habilitation of patients identified with balance system dysfunction.

"Balance system assessment" refers to a series of procedures designed to evaluate patients presenting with dizziness and/or imbalance. These procedures enable the practitioner to detect and monitor dysfunction within the vestibular, visual and soma to sensory systems of balance-disordered.

Reference this material as follows: American Speech-Language-Hearing Association (1992). Balance System Assessment ASHA (March, Suppl. 7), 9–12, patients, and in some cases, provide suggestions for (re)habilitation to the appropriate personnel.

III. Purpose

Although it is recognized that not all audiologists are or will be involved in the assessment of balance-disordered patients, this document provides guidelines for those audiologists who are or may be involved. The purpose of this position statement is to: (a) inform audiologists that performing balance assessment procedures is within the scope of practice of audiology; (b) identify the collection of procedures known as balance system assessment; (c) advise audiologists of the education, training, circumstances, and precautions that should be considered prior to undertaking the procedures; (d) provide guidance for audiologists as to the knowledge and skills that are required to perform balance system assessment; and (e) ultimately, to educate healthcare professionals, consumers, and members of the general public of the services offered by audiologists as qualified healthcare providers.

The spirit of this document is not to mandate a single method of education and training. The intention is to delineate the role of audiologists related to balance system assessment and to suggest minimum knowledge and skills required to begin work in this area.

IV. Scope of Practice

It is the position of the American Speech-Language-Hearing Association (ASHA) that balance system assessment is within the scope of practice of audiologists. Practice in this area requires that audiologists possess sufficient knowledge and skills to conduct and interpret the range of vestibular, ocular motor, and balance function tests (Cyr, 11-991; Kileny, 1985; Stockwell, 1986; Stockwell, 1990). Audiologists should possess knowledge of anatomy, physiology, and pathophysiology of the balance and auditory systems, medical conditions that affect test results, electrophysiological and biomedical techniques, management of sick patients in accordance with local medical policy, and physical or occupational therapy procedures related to the assessment and (re)habilitation of balance-disordered patients (Shepard, Telian, & Smith-Wheelock, 1990). In addition, clinical experience and proficiency in the conduct of basic and advanced balance test procedures are required.

It is noted that the level of experience, skills, and knowledge may differ greatly among audiologists working actively in the area of balance assessment. It is recognized that other professions or related fields also may be involved with assessment and/or (re)habilitation of balance-disordered patients. As a result, there is no intention to exclude or influence their participation. This document recognizes further that the area of balance system assessment is changing rapidly and there is no intention to preclude future procedures within the scope of practice.

If practitioners choose to perform these procedures, indicators should be developed, as part of a continuous quality improvement process, to monitor and evaluate the appropriateness, efficacy, and safety of the procedure conducted.

V. Education and Training

Depending on factors such as individual job setting, local practice policy and the type of vestibular/balance assessment procedures available, audiologists may function on a continuum from basic test administration through test interpretation. As a result, education and training may vary. Education should be obtained through the audiologist's academic program or through a clinical program structured to cover all aspects of balance assessment. Training should take place in a clinical setting affiliated with medical personnel and should include exposure to a number of diverse patients. In addition, all practitioners must determine whether or not they have obtained a sufficient degree of education and training to be competent to perform and interpret the various tests of balance function.

VI. Precautions

Patient: Some procedures may result in patient discomfort or adverse reactions. It is the responsibility of practitioners who conduct or supervise such procedures to develop specific protocols in conjuction with appropriate medical personnel to ensure patient safety and comfort.

The protocols should address:

1. Facilities, equipment, and protocols necessary to perform the tests in a safe and comfortable manner;
2. Identification of personnel responsible for the tests;
3. Identification of appropriate medical personnel to contact in the event that emergency medical assistance is needed;
4. Informed consent, including known risks of the tests, in conjuction with institutional and/or regulatory bodies;
5. Documentation of patient condition before, during, and following the tests.

Practitioner: Some procedures may introduce the possibility of practitioner exposure to bloodborne pathogens. It is recommended that the practitioner follow the Universal Precautions contained in the Center for Disease Control Morbidity and Mortality Weekly Report (Perspectives in Disease Prevention and Health Promotion, June 24, 1988. Vol.37, No.24:377–388) or ASHA AIDS/ HIV Update (ASHA, 1990). In addition, practitioners must determine the potential professional liability for any procedure they conduct or supervise. Institutional and/or regulatory bodies, such as state licensure boards, should be informed about these procedures as within the scope of practice. In addition, they should be consulted to determine policies related to professional responsibility and liability, and to ensure that there are no limitations imposed on the scope of audiology practice that restricts the performance of these procedures or their insurance coverage.

VII. Definitions

"Balance assessment" refers to the evaluation of vestibular and extravestibular (visual and somatosensory) systems using a variety of vestibular or balance tests. Those tests include but are not limited to electronystagmography (ENG), rotation and posturography. Electronystagmography includes tests of the gaze, optokinetic, ocular saccade and pursuit systems, spontaneous, positional and positioning nystagmus, and caloric irrigation. Tests of rotation might include the rotary chair test (sinusoidal, pseudo-random, off-axis, low and high frequency) or auto-rotation test. Posturography includes static and dynamic conditions along with accessory tests (ear canal pressure, EMG recording, etc.).

"Balance (re)habilitation" refers to nonmedical therapy for balance-disordered patients. Audiologists working with such patients should be aware of the various (re)habilitative therapies employed. It is not the intent of these guidelines to prepare audiologists for the (re)habilitative aspects of balance dysfunction. However, based on their training background and experience, they should be prepared to use their knowledge of balance system assessment for the purpose of interacting with rehabilitation professionals (when appropriate) by integrating balance test results in (re)habilitation programs.

VIII. Knowledge and Skills

All audiologists who intend to perform these procedures must ensure that they have acquired the knowledge and skills necessary to do so accurately and effectively. Outlined below are objectives and the basic knowledge and skill necessary to become proficient in balance system assessment techniques.

A. Objective: To conduct calibration and function checks on equipment.
    Knowledge/skills needed:
    1. Knowledge of general electrophysiological techniques and bioelectrical recording procedures.
    2. Fundamental and practical knowledge of electronic instrumentation used in eye movement recording procedures.
B. Objective: To develop normative values for each test administered, when necessary.
    Knowledge/skills needed:
    1. Familiarity with and proficiency in performing each individual test.
    2. Knowledge of basic statistical design.
C. Objective: To administer routine vestibular and ocular motor tests and possess the ability to change the test protocol when required.
    Knowledge/skills needed:
    1. Efficiency in performing the ENG test battery. Sufficient practicum should have been obtained on a number of patients, preferably during graduate training.
    2. Knowledge of the theory and rationale for each ENG subtest.
    3. Understanding of the interaction between each subtest and the medical conditions which may affect or alter the conduct of the tests or the results generated. Knowledge of other factors that may affect test results. (e.g., patient alertness and medication).
    4. Knowledge of anatomy and physiology related to the type of eye movement recording and the system(s) being evaluated by each type.
    5. Knowledge of patient preparation including placing electrodes, verifying electrode contact, and providing clear and accurate patient instructions
D. Objective: To conduct otoscopic examinations (governed by local policy and training) to note cerumen obstruction and tympanic membrane integrity.
    Knowledge/skills needed:
    1. Refer to ASHA Position Statement and Guidelines on External Auditory Canal Examination and Cerumen Management.

E.   Objective: To integrate all test results incorporating patient history, symptoms, and other pertinent information into reports with recommendations.

Knowledge/skills needed:

1. Knowledge of anatomy, physiology, and pathophysiology of the balance system. This might include, but not be limited to the vestibular, vestibular-ocular, vestibular-spinal, visual and somatosensory systems, both peripheral and central, sensory and motor.
2. Knowledge of the physiological and functional interaction among these systems.
3. General medical background related to various conditions and events affecting the balance systems and the tests designed to evaluate those systems. This might include, but not be limited to, the effects of medication or specific medical entities causing test artifacts, such as extra-ocular muscle weakness, mental or emotional status of the patient, orthopedic or neurological deficits, and so forth. Exposure to medical specialties such as otolaryngology, neurology, and physical medicine is suggested.
4. Knowledge and skill related balance assessment procedures, both basic (ENG) and advanced (rotation and posturography), and an understanding of the interaction between test results and patient symptoms. Sufficient practicum should be obtained during their graduate program or at a 'Center of Excellence' to prepare audiologists both for test administration and interpretation.

F.   Objective: To develop protocols for management of sick patients in conjuction with appropriate medical personnel.

Knowledge/skills needed:

1. Demonstration of current certification in CPR and other lifesaving procedures (Basic Life Support) for adult and pediatric patients.
2. Knowledge of general medical conditions that may be present during the course of the testing.

G.   Objective: To interact with appropriate rehabilitation personnel (when appropriate) for the development of rehabilitation programs for balance-disordered patients.

Knowledge/skills needed:

1. Knowledge of therapy approaches and techniques as they relate to (re)habilitation of balance-disordered patients.
2. Knowledge and understanding of the functional impact of vestibular and extra-vestibular system dysfunction of balance and equilibrium.

References

American Speech-Language-Hearing Association. (1990, December). Report Update. AIDS/HIV: Implications for speech-language pathologists and audiologists. ASHA, 32, 46–48.

Centers for Disease Control. (1988). Morbidity and Mortality weekly report: Perspectives in disease prevention and health promotion. CDC, 37, 377–388.

Cyr, D.G. (1990). Vestibular system assessment. In W. Rintelmann (Ed.), Hearing assessment, (pp. 739–803). Austin, TX: Pro-Ed.

Kileny, P. (1985). Evaluation of vestibular function. In J. Katz (Ed.), Handbook of clinical audiology, (pp. 582–603). Baltimore, MD: Williams & Wilkins.

Martin, F., & Morris, L. (1989). Current audiological practices in the United States. The Hearing Journal, 25–44.

Shepard, N., Telian, S., & Smith-Wheelock, M. (1990, May). Habilitation and balance retraining therapy: A retrospective review. Neurology Clinic of North America, 459–475.

Stockwell, C. (1986). Vestibular function tests. In C.W. Cummings (ed.). Otolaryngology head and neck surgery, 4 (pp. 2743–2763). St. Louis, MO: C.V. Mosby.

Stockwell, C. (1990). Vestibular function testing: 4-year update. In C.W. Cummings (Ed.). Otolaryngology head and neck surgery. Update II, (pp. 39–53). St. Louis, MO: C.V. Mosby.

Audiology statement.

ASHA Scope of Practice in Audiology (1996)

"Preamble: Audiologists provide comprehensive diagnostic and rehabilitative services for all areas of auditory, vestibular, and related disorders."

ASHA Definition of an Audiologist

Audiologists are autonomous professionals who identify, assess, and manage disorders of the auditory, balance and other neural systems.... Audiologists are involved in auditory and related research pertinent to the prevention, identification, and management of hearing loss, tinnitus, and balance system dysfunction.
    The practice of audiology includes the following:

1. Activities that identify, assess, diagnose, manage, and interpret test results related to disorders of human hearing, balance, and other neural systems
2. Otoscopic examination and external canal management for removal of cerumen in order to evaluate hearing or balance
3. The conduct and interpretation of behavioral, electroacoustic, or electrophysiologic methods used to assess hearing, balance, and neural system function and provision of rehabilitation to persons with balance disorders using habituation, exercise therapy, and balance retraining
4. Consultation to individuals, public and private agencies, and governmental bodies, or as an expert witness regarding legal interpretations of audiology findings, effects of hearing loss and balance system disorders, and relevant noise-related considerations

Outcomes of Audiology Services

The following listing describes the types of outcomes that consumers may expect to receive from an audiologist.

1. Identification of populations and individuals with or at risk of balance disorders
2. Counseling regarding the effects of balance system dysfunction (www.ASHA.org)

ASHA has also issued position statements on "Balance System Assessment" and Vestibular Rehabilitation:

The American Academy of Audiology (AAA) has not issued any specific position statement regarding the management of patients with vestibular dysfunction; however, their scope of practice statement dictates that all facets of assessment and treatment of patients with vestibular function are within the scope of practice for audiologists.

Audiology: Scope of Practice

AAA Definition of an Audiologist

An audiologist is a person who, by virtue of academic degree, clinical training, and licensed to practice and/or professional credential, is uniquely qualified to provide a comprehensive array of professional; services related to the assessment and habilitation/rehabilitation of persons with auditory and vestibular impairments, and to the prevention of these impairments.... In addition, professional activities related to assessment and rehabilitation of persons with vestibular disorders are within the scope of practice of audiologists.

AAA Scope of Practice

The scope of practice of audiologists is defined by training and knowledge base of professionals who are licensed or credentialed to practice as audiologists. Areas of practice include assessment and habilitation/rehabilitation of individuals with auditory and vestibular disorders, prevention of hearing loss, and research in normal and disordered auditory and vestibular function.

Assessment

Assessment of the vestibular system includes administration and interpretation of clinical and electrophysiologic tests of equilibrium. Assessment is accomplished using standardized testing procedures and appropriately calibrated instrumentation.

Habilitation and Rehabilitation

Audiologists are also involved in the rehabilitation of persons with vestibular disorders. They participate as full members of vestibular rehabilitation teams to recommend and carry out goals of vestibular rehabilitation therapy including, for example, habituation exercises, balance retraining exercises, and general conditioning exercises (www.audiology.org).

Role of Physical Therapy

Physical therapists (PTs) have traditionally taken the lead role in providing ongoing rehabilitation to patients with vestibular dysfunction or nonvestibular balance problems. Several causes of dysequilibrium and gait disorders, such as peripheral neuropathy and musculoskeletal injuries, fall squarely in the realm of physical therapy. Most PTs, as part of their basic training, learn to deal with these types of disorders. Some PTs with additional experience and training may become involved in the evaluation and treatment of vestibular disorders. Box 7–2 is a reprint of a recent scope of practice statement from the American Physical Therapy Association (APTA, 1997).

Box 7–2

Model Definition of Physical Therapy for State Practice Acts
[BOD 02-97-03-06; Amended BOD 03-95-24-64, BOD 06-94-03-04, BOD 03-93-18-46]
Physical therapy, which is the care and services provided by or under the direction and supervision of a physical therapist, includes the following:
1. Examining (history, systems review, and tests and measures) individuals with impairment, functional limitation, and disability or other health-related conditions to determine a diagnosis, prognosis, and intervention; tests and measures may include the following:
- Aerobic capacity and endurance
- Anthropometric characteristics
- Arousal, mentation, and cognition
- Assistive and adaptive devices
- Community and work (job/school/play) integration or reintegration
- Cranial nerve integrity
- Ergonomics and body mechanics
- Gait, locomotion, and balance
- Integumentary integrity
- Joint integrity and mobility
- Motor function
- Muscle performance
- Neuromotor development and sensory integration
- Orthotic, protective, and supportive devices
- Pain
- Posture
- Prosthetic requirements
- Range of motion
- Reflex integrity
- Self-care and home management
- Sensory integrity

- Ventilation, respiration, and circulation

2. Alleviating impairment and functional limitation by designing, implementing, and modifying therapeutic interventions that may include, but are not limited to:
- Coordination, communication, and documentation
- Patient/client-related instruction
- Therapeutic exercise (include aerobic conditioning)
- Functional training in self-care and home management (including activities of daily living and instrumental activities of daily living)
- Functional training in community and work (job/school/play) integration or reintegration activities (including instrumental activities of daily living, work hardening, and work conditioning)
- Manual therapy techniques (including mobilization and manipulation)
- Prescription, application, and, as appropriate, fabrication of assistive, adaptive, orthotic, protective, supportive, and prosthetic devices and equipment
- Airway clearance techniques
- Wound management
- Electrotherapeutic modalities
- Physical agents and mechanical modalities

3. Preventing injury, impairment, functional limitation, and disability, including the promotion and maintenance of fitness, health, and quality of life in all age populations

4. Engaging in consultation, education, and research

Role of Support Personnel

The rising costs of health care have made it essential that services be provided in the most cost-effective manner. The use of support personnel can allow the professional to practice more effectively and increase the number of patients seen in a given period. The obvious concern over the use of support personnel is whether they are qualified to provide tasks assigned by the professional. Both ASHA and the APTA have issued statements regarding minimal training and supervision requirements for support personnel in the fields of audiology and physical therapy.

Position Statement and Guidelines on Support Personnel in Audiology

This policy document of the American Speech-Language-Hearing Association (ASHA) reflects the Association's position that the Certificate of Clinical Competence-Audiology (CCC-A) is a nationally recognized quality indicator and education standard for the profession. The following statement includes the CCC-A as the appropriate credential for audiologists supervising support personnel. The consensus panel document's exclusion of the CCC-A conflicts with ASHA's policy.

Member organizations that composed the consensus panel on support personnel in audiology included: Academy of Dispensing Audiologists (ADA), American Academy of Audiology (AAA), ASHA, Educational Audiology Association (EAA), Military Audiology Association (MAA), and the National Hearing Conservation Association (NHCA). Representatives to the panel included Donald Bender (AAA) and Evelyn Cherow (ASHA), co-chairs; James McDonald and Meredy Hase (ADA); Albert deChiccis and Cheryl deConde Johnson (AAA); Chris Halpin and Deborah Price (ASHA); Peggy Benson (EAA); James Jerome (MAA); and Lloyd Bowling and Richard Danielson (NHCA).

ASHA's Legislative Council and Executive Board elected not to adopt the consensus panel document, because it excluded the CCC-A. In all other aspects, the documents remain similar. This position statement and guidelines supersede the audiology sections of the Guidelines for the Employment and Utilization of Supportive Personnel (LC 32–80).

Reference this material as: American Speech-Language-Hearing Association. (1998). Position statement and guidelines on support personnel in audiology. *Asha*, 40 (Suppl. 18), pp. 19–21

Index terms: audiological support personnel, audiology technicians, paraprofessionals, supervision, support personnel, technicians

I. Introduction

Federal and state health care and education reform initiatives, changing U.S. demographics, and the broadening scope of practice of audiologists (ASHA, 1996; Educational Testing Service, 1995; AAA, 1993) have affected the delivery of audiology services. Audiologists are using support personnel in audiology service delivery systems to ensure both the accessibility and the highest quality of audiology care while addressing productivity and cost-benefit concerns. In an analysis of state licensure laws (Larson & Lynch, 1995), ASHA found that in the 45 states that regulate one or both professions of audiology and speech-language pathology, 30 recognize support personnel; 22 states have promulgated rules regulating support personnel in all work settings and 5 were in process of creating these rules. This position statement and guidelines do not supersede federal legislation and regulation requirements, any existing state licensure laws, or affect the interpretation or implementation of such laws. The document may serve, however, as a guide for the development of new laws or, at the appropriate lime, for revising existing licensure laws.

II. Position Statement

It is the position of ASHA that support personnel may assist audiologists in delivery of serviced where appropriate. The roles and tasks of audiology support personnel will be assigned only by supervising audiologists. Supervising audiologists will provide appropriate training that is competency-based and specific to job performance. Supervision will be comprehensive, periodic, and documented. The supervising audiologist maintains the legal and ethical responsibilities for all assigned audiology activities provided by support personnel. The needs of the consumer of audiology services and protection of that consumer will always be paramount (ASHA, 1996; ASHA, 1994: AAA, 1996–97: NHCA, 1995). Audiologists are uniquely educated and specialized in the diagnosis and rehabilitation of hearing and related disorders. As such, audiologists are the appropriate, qualified professionals to hire, supervise, and train audiology support personnel.

III. Guidelines

Definitions

> *Support personnel*: People who, after appropriate training, perform tasks that are prescribed, directed, and supervised by an audiologist.
>
> *Supervising audiologist*: An audiologist who has attained license (where applicable), holds certification (CCC-A) from the American Speech-Language-Hearing Association, and who has been practicing for at least one year after meeting these requirements.

Qualifications for Support Personnel

1. Have a high school degree or equivalent.
2. Have communication and interpersonal skills necessary for the tasks assigned.
3. Have a basic understanding of the needs of the population being served.
4. Have net training requirements and have competency-based skills necessary to the performance of specific assigned tasks.
5. Have any additional qualifications established by the supervising audiologist to meet the specific needs of the audiology program and the population being served.

Training for Support Personnnel

Training for support personnel should be well defined and specific to the assigned task(s). The supervising audiologist will ensure that the scope and intensity of training encompass all of the activities assigned to the support personnel. Training should be competency-based and provided through a variety of formal and informal instructional methods. Audiologists should provide support personnel with information on roles and functions. Continuing opportunities should be provided to ensure that practices are current and that skills are maintained. The supervising audiologist will maintain written documentation of training activities.

Role of Support Personnel

Audiology support personnel may engage in only those tasks that are planned, delegated, and supervised by the audiologist. The specific roles of audiology support personnel will be influenced by the particular needs of the audiologist and must be determined by the audiologist responsible for the support personnel's training and supervision.

Audiology support personnel will not engage independently in the following activities. This list provides examples and is not intended to be all-inclusive.

- Interpreting observations or data into diagnostic statements of clinical management strategies or procedures.
- Determining case selection.
- Transmitting clinical information, either verbally or in writing, to anyone without the approval of the supervising audiologist.
- Composing clinical reports except for progress notes to be reviewed by the audiologist and held in the patient's/client's records.
- Referring a patient/client to other professionals or agencies.
- Referring to him or her either orally or in writing with a title other than one determined by the supervising audiologist.
- Signing any formal documents (e.g., treatment plans, reimbursement forms, or reports).
- Discharging a patient/client from services.
- Communicating with the patient/client, family, or others regarding any aspect of patient/client status or service without the specific consent of the supervising audiologist.

Supervision of Support Personnel

Supervising audiologists will have the primary role in all administrative actions related to audiology support personnel, such as hiring, training, determining competency, and conducting performance evaluations. In addition, the supervising audiologist maintains final approval of all directives given by administrators and other professionals regarding audiology tasks.

Supervising audiologists will assign specific tasks to the support person. Such tasks must not require the exercise of professional judgement or entail interpretation of results or the development or modification of treatment plans.

The amount and type of supervision required should be based on skills and experience of the support person, the needs of patients/clients served, the service-delivery setting, the tasks assigned, and other factors. For example, more intense supervision will be required during orientation of a new support person; initiation of a new program, task, or equipment; or a change in patient/client status.

The number of support personnel supervised by a given audiologist must be consistent with the delivery of appropriate, quality service. It is the responsibility of the individual supervisor to protect the interests of patients/clients in a manner consistent with state licensure requirements, where applicable, and the ASHA Code of Ethics.

References

American Academy of Audiology. (1991, Jan.–Feb.). Audiology: Scope of practice. *Audiology Today,* 5(1), 16–17.

American Speech-Language-Hearing Association. (1998, March), *Code of ethics. Asha,* 40 (Suppl. 18), 43–45.

American Speech-Language-Hearing Association. (1996, Spring), Scope of practice in audiology. *Asha,* 38 (Suppl. 16), 12–14.

American Academy of Audiology. (1996), *Code of Ethics.* McLean, VA: Author.

Educational Testing Service. (1995). *The practice of audiology: A study of clinical activities and knowledge areas for the certified audiologist.* Rockville, MD: American Speech-Language-Hearing Association.

Larson, S., & Lynch, U. (1995). *Report; State, regulation of audiology and speech-language pathology support personnel.* Rockville, MD: American Speech-Language-Hearing Association. Unpublished manuscript.

National Hearing Conservation Association. (1995). *Code of ethics.* Milwaukee, WT: Author.

(American Speech Language Association, 1998)

Physical Therapist Assistants

The PT assistant is an educated health care provider who assists the PT in the provision of physical therapy. The PT assistant is a graduate of an associate degree program for PT assistants that is accredited by an agency recognized by the Commission on Accreditation in Physical Therapy Education (CAPTE).

The PT of record is the person who is directly responsible for the actions of the PT assistant. The PT assistant may perform physical therapy procedures and related tasks that have been selected and delegated by the supervising PT. Where permitted by law, the PT assistant also may carry out routine operational functions, including the supervision of the physical therapy aide and documentation of progress. The ability of the PT assistant to perform the selected and delegated tasks should be assessed on an ongoing basis by the supervising PT. The PT assistant may modify a specific intervention procedure in accordance with changes in patient–client status and within the scope of the established plan of care.

Physical Therapy Aides

The physical therapy aide is a nonlicensed worker who is specifically trained under the direction of a PT. The physical therapy aide performs designated routine tasks related to the operation of a physical therapy service delegated by the PT or, in accordance with the law, by a PT assistant.

The PT of record is the person who is directly responsible for the actions of the physical therapy aide. The physical therapy aide provides support that may include patient-related and non-patient–related duties. The physical therapy aide functions only with the continuous on-site supervision of the PT or, where allowable by law or regulation, the PT assistant. Continuous on-site supervision requires the presence of the PT assistant in the immediate areas.

Other Support Personnel

When other personnel (e.g., exercise physiologists, athletic trainers, massage therapists) work within the supervision of a physical therapy service, they should be employed under the appropriate title. Any involvement in the patient–client care activities should be within the limits of their education, in accordance with the applicable laws and regulations, and at the discretion of the PT. If such personnel function as an extension of the physical therapist's license, however, their title and all services that they provide must be in accordance with state and federal laws and regulations (American Physical Therapy Association, 1997).

References

American Academy of Neurology. (1996). Assessment: Electronystagmography. *Neurology*, *46*, 1763–1766.

American Academy of Otolaryngology-Head and Neck Surgery. (2000). Clinical indicators compendium: Canalith repositioning. *Bulletin*, *19*(6), 50.

American Academy of Otolaryngology–Head and Neck Surgery. (1998). Dynamic posturography and vestibular testing. *Bulletin*, *17*(10), 12.

American Academy of Otolaryngology–Head and Neck Surgery. (1998). The scope of Otolaryngology. *Bulletin*, *17*(10), 19.

American Academy of Otolaryngology–Head and Neck Surgery. (1998). Vestibular rehabilitation / balance retraining Therapy. *Bulletin*, *17*(10), 20.

American Physical Therapy Association. (1997). Guide to physical therapist practice. *J Am Phys Ther Assoc 77*(11), 1155–1674.

American Speech, Language and Hearing Association (ASHA) Ad Hoc Committee on Vestibular Rehabilitation. (1999). Role of audiologists in vestibular and balance rehabilitation: Position statement, guidelines, and technical report. *ASHA*, *41*(2), 13–22.

American Speech, Language and Hearing Association (ASHA). (1998). Position statement and guidelines on support personnel in audiology. *ASHA*, *40*(2), 19–21.

American Speech-Language Hearing Association (ASHA). (1992). Balance system assessment. *ASHA*, *7*, 9–12.

Givens, G. (1994). The profession, licensure, and evolution of practice. *Sem Hear*, *15*(3), 175–177.

Goebel, J. (1992). Training the balance specialist [Editorial]. *Am J Otol*, *13*(1), 2.

Kroenke, K., Hoffman, R., & Einstadter, D. (2000). How common are various causes of dizziness? *South Med J*, *93*(2), 160–167.

Kroenke, K., Lucas, C., Rosenberg, M., Scherokman, B., Herbers, J., Wehrle, P., & Boggi, J. (1992). Causes of persistent dizziness: A prospective study of 100 patients in ambulatory care. *Ann Intern Med*, *17*(11), 898–904.

Lawson, J., Fitzgerald, J., Birchall, J., Aldren, C. P., & Kenny, R. A. (1999). Diagnosis of geriatric patients with severe dizziness. *J Am Geriatr Soc*, *47*, 12–17.

Martin, F., Champlin, C., & Chambers, J. (1998). Seventh survey of audiometric practices in the United States. *J Am Acad Audiol*, *9*(2), 95–104.

Sloane, P. D., Hartman, M., & Mitchell, C. M. (1994) Psychological factors associated with Chronic dizziness in patients aged 60 and over. *J Am Geriatr Soc*, *42*, 847-853.

Turner, R. (1992). Autonomy (editorial). *Am J Audiol*, *1*(3), 2.

8

Marketing and Financial Aspects

Marketing Aspects

"If you build it, they will come."

This line is the mantra from the movie "Field of Dreams" starring Kevin Costner in which a voice from above commanded him to build a baseball field. Costner's character in the movie had to have enough faith to build the field in hopes of saving his failing farm from bank foreclosure. Health care practitioners (HCPs) must have more than faith when making decisions about starting or expanding their practice. No longer can HCPs simply "hang up their shingle" and expect to succeed in today's marketplace. The provision of health care has become much more complicated and competitive. Nearly all potential patients have some type of health insurance, such as Medicare, Medicaid, or private insurance. Many are members of health maintenance organizations (HMOs), which can influence the patient's choice of services and providers. Marketing and negotiating contracts are critical to the success of most health care practices as medicine enters the twenty-first century.

Health care has improved in many ways. Some of these changes have benefited primarily the patient while at the same time making it more difficult for the HCP to succeed financially. Improvements in technology and the sheer amount of information now available are too much for one person to learn. HCPs have been forced to specialize to be current with the ever-advancing fund of medical information. As a result patient expectations are higher, and the responsible HCP understands that this restricts the types of patients he or she should be treating. A second factor (although not true of all specialties) is the oversupply of physicians in many areas. Over the past 30 years, the supply of physicians in the United States has grown at a rate three times faster than the general population (Brown & Morley, 1986). Government intervention in health care and cost-saving attempts from HMOs have resulted in restricted and reduced reimbursement for many HCPs.

Historically, marketing has been regarded as distasteful and even unethical by some medical societies. Some professionals view marketing simply as advertising and believe that marketing undermines the integrity of their profession. Although advertising may be a component of a marketing plan, marketing should be viewed as a method of presenting oneself to the public in a way that improves the image of the practice, and it makes the public aware of the services offered. To paraphrase a common marketing slogan,"It doesn't matter how good your product or services are if no one knows they are available."

Marketing involves making decisions regarding the four Ps:

1. Product (or service)
2. Place
3. Promotion
4. Pricing

Product refers to the specific product or service that is being offered. While on initial inspection it would appear that the product being offered at a multi-disciplinary balance clinic would be the evaluation and treatment of vestibular and related disorders, from a marketing perspective the product differs depending on the consumer. Patients suffering from dizziness and dysequilibrium are interested in a correct diagnosis; a reduction of symptoms; and an increase in mobility, independence, and quality of life. Managed care companies are interested in practices that can reduce their cost of caring for patients with dizziness and dysequilibrium. Hospitals and other employers of HCPs providing these services are interested in increasing their revenue and prestige.

Place refers to the location of the practice. A balance clinic situated close to a major university medical center offering vestibular diagnostics is not likely to flourish. On the other extreme, a clinic in a sparsely populated area may find it difficult to develop an adequate patient load even in the absence of competition. The nature of a multidisciplinary clinic and the size and cost of required equipment restrict the option of multiple offices. One well-known vestibular clinic has a van equipped with full electronystagmography (ENG) equipment, and a technician drives around the region performing ENG examinations in several physicians' offices. Most professionals need to decide on a location that is accessible to both the public and convenient for members of the multidisciplinary team.

Promotion includes any methods used to provide information to the public. Promotions can take the form of paid advertisements, newsletters, speeches, phone solicitations, or free screenings. In medical practices, a commonly used and effective method of promotion is personal contact with potential referring physicians.

Pricing is probably the most complicated of the four Ps as it applies to the delivery of health care. In most businesses, the laws of supply and demand determine pricing. For the most part, payments for health care services are determined by a third party and do not reflect any increase for increased demand for the service; therefore, the HCP must control costs to ensure that the services provided allow for some profit at the current reimbursement rate.

Marketing to Physicians

Chapter 1 of this book outlines the primary care physicians' (PCP) approach to treating patients complaining of dizziness. The gap between "what works," and "what is done" is significant. A lag of several years occurs from the time a clinical study demonstrates the effectiveness of a particular treatment and the time the new treatment is put into practice in the most medical practices (Antman, Lau, Kupelnick, Mosteller, & Chalmers, 1992). PCPs are obviously interested in the best care for their patients, but many are unaware of diagnostic and treatment techniques available today. The key to marketing to physicians resides in education, which can be accomplished by many of the promotion techniques already mentioned. Physician newsletters (see Appendix E) covering topics related to vestibular function (as well as any other services offered by the practice) can be mailed to local physicians' offices. Mailing lists can often be obtained by the local hospital or medical society.

Personal contact with potential referring physicians allows an informal way to let them know about a practice as well as the personal philosophies and interests of the staff. Because most physicians are very busy, offering to bring lunch for the physician and staff could provide a relaxed atmosphere and an enthusiastic welcome from the staff. This technique has been used successfully by pharmaceutical representatives for years in an effort to obtain "face time" with the physician.

An effective method of educating physicians is by doing continuing medical education (CME) seminars for the local hospital or medical society. The seminar does not need to be extremely detailed but should allow the physician to understand more clearly what type of patients can benefit from being referred to a balance clinic and what will happen once the patients get there (Table 8–1). Be prepared to back up any statements made by citing published clinical studies, and remember that the current thinking regarding treating vestibular disorders is almost 180 degrees in opposition to the methods (vestibular suppressant medication) used by many PCPs.

Physicians, like all people, are creatures of habit. Whereas physicians may understand the benefits of referring a patient to a balance clinic, this requires an alteration in their practice habits. Making a referral as easy as possible will likely increase the number of referrals. Providing a clear and concise referral sheet will make the referral process easier (see Appendix F). By providing a checklist on the referral sheet, a great deal can be learned about the patient's medical history and reason for the referral with minimal time output on the part of the referring physician. The referral sheet should also offer the referring physician the opportunity to participate in the disposition of the patient once a diagnosis is obtained. Many specialists (otolaryngologists and neurologists) may wish to handle treatment themselves. Primary care and unrelated specialists often prefer the balance clinic to assume care of the patient in relation to their vestibular related complaints. It is essential that the referring physician be given this choice and that the balance clinic staff respects the choice.

A frequently encountered problem is the handling of patients who are referred for immediate or emergent evaluation. Patients with acute vertigo and ataxia require immediate evaluation. Patients with chronic complaints of recurrent

Table 8–1. Outline of a Continuing Medical Education Program on the Evaluation and Treatment of Dizziness

---

1. Demographics. Although most practicing physicians will have an opinion about the prevalence of dizziness, epidemiologic data are always helpful in supporting the need for professional services.

2. Consequences and Costs. The costs associated with falls and hip fractures are staggering. It has been demonstrated that physicians often underestimate the negative effect of vestibular disorders on the patient's quality of life (Honrubia, Bell, Harris, Baloh, & Fisher, 1996).

3. Terminology. Brief definitions of vestibular-related terms allow the physician to understand more clearly the remainder of the presentation.

4. Anatomy and Physiology. A brief presentation of the role and function of the vestibular ocular reflex and balance in general allows the physician to understand more clearly the source of symptoms and the purpose of specific vestibular and balance tests.

5. Common Vestibular Disorders. Detailed descriptions of associated symptoms and brief descriptions of pathophysiology will help the physician to recognize potential patients for the balance clinic.

6. Nonvestibular Disorders. Discussing conditions such as orthostatic hypotension and hyperventilation, which often present as complaints of dizziness, will allow the physician to make more appropriate referrals.

7. Screening Techniques. This information helps the physician to determine which patients require additional evaluation.

8. Diagnostic Tests Performed in the Balance Clinic. The physician must understand what information can be provided by the balance clinic to understand the value of these services.

9. Treatment Techniques. The concept of vestibular rehabilitation is foreign to many primary care physicians. By explaining the process of central compensation, physicians can better understand the possible negative effects of overuse of vestibular-suppressant medication.

10. Outcome Measures. The ability to demonstrate benefit from services provided may help in overcoming skepticism regarding a recommended change in the approach to treating patients complaining of dizziness.

---

vertigo or dysequilibrium often require extensive, time-consuming examination, which presents a problem when patients with chronic complaints are referred on an emergent basis. Again, the solution to this problem is education of the referring physician. Through screening techniques covered in Chapter 3, the referring physician should be able to make appropriate referrals. To avoid alienating the referring physician, the scheduling personnel should be instructed to work in any patients that complain of acute vertigo or ataxia. A brief examination to rule out neurologic emergencies or to treat the patient symptomatically can usually be accomplished in just a few minutes. Further evaluation and follow-up can be scheduled for a later date. From a marketing standpoint, refusing to see a patient because the clinic schedule is full is a luxury that a practice hoping to grow cannot afford.

Marketing to Hospital Administrators

Hospital administrators may be motivated by three factors:

1. The "bottom-line" or financial well-being of the hospital
2. The quality of care offered by the hospital
3. The prestige of being considered a top hospital in the area

A successful multidisciplinary balance clinic associated with a hospital can contribute to all three of these motivating factors and may put the members of the balance clinic in a position to negotiate some assistance in developing and marketing their services.

At this time, balance clinics are still relatively rare and are not found in most communities. This means that a successful balance clinic will likely draw patients from a wider geographic region than most services offered by the hospital. This will result in an increase in associated services such as imaging, laboratory work, and referrals to physical therapy and other specialists associated with the hospital. Once patients become familiar with the location and staff at the hospital, they may elect to travel a little farther for future medical needs.

Hospitals, like physicians, are often concerned with the content of advertisements designed to promote their facility. The addition and promotion of a new service such as a balance clinic give the hospital a reason to put their name out in front of the public. The exposure is good for the hospital and allows the hospital to inform the public of a service that may not be available at surrounding hospitals. The balance clinic may be able to negotiate a marketing budget to be covered by the hospitals' marketing department.

Marketing to the Public

Vestibular disorders can have a significant negative impact on quality of life. As mentioned earlier, physicians often underestimate this impact on the patient (Honrubia et al., 1996). As a result, patients may feel frustrated and begin to seek solutions on their own. Providing information directly to the public is an important method of marketing the balance clinic. A word of caution: A significant number of patients complaining of dizziness may have medical problems that cannot be addressed in a balance clinic. Offering direct access to the clinic without prior primary care medical screening can result in a potentially dangerous and libelous situation.

WORD OF MOUTH

Satisfied patients are the strongest marketing tool a practice can have. Staab (2000) reports that 68% of patients (customers) discontinue to patronize a business because of "an attitude of indifference" by someone in the office. The importance of "good" word of mouth is outlined by Hosford-Dunn, Dunn, & Harford (1995) based on a publication by Boyet and Conn (1991) that lists the findings of surveys completed by the Technical Assistance Research Programs in Washington, D.C.

- Consumers were five times more likely to stop doing business with a company for poor service than for poor product quality or high cost.
- Ninety-six percent of a company's dissatisfied customers never complained to the company, but 90% quit doing business with the company.
- Almost all customers (95%) with a complaint will stay with the company if their complaint is resolved quickly.
- The average dissatisfied customer complains about the company to nine other people; 13% complain to at least 20 people.
- A customer who is pleased with a company will tell five other people. Many of these people will become customers of the company.
- The cost of losing a customer is five times the annual value of the customer's account.
- Improving quality of service is much more cost-effective than other promotional efforts: It costs five times as much to obtain a customer than to keep one.

Many factors can increase patient satisfaction and, it is hoped, improve "word-of-mouth" marketing potential. Obviously, the correct diagnosis and effective treatment of a chronic balance disorder will do more than anything else to increase patient satisfaction. Because of this, adequate diagnostic facilities and training are imperative. As in any business or medical practice, there is a learning curve that requires a certain amount of time and experience before competency is achieved. Marketing one's practice as a specialty clinic for balance disorders brings with it the responsibility of dealing with unusual presentations of vestibular disorders as well as the responsibility of recognizing an emergent condition requiring referral for appropriate care. From a marketing standpoint, even a relatively harmless error or oversight can prove devastating to the reputation of a new clinic.

Improved communication with patients will increase overall satisfaction. Patients are often frightened and uncomfortable when undergoing medical examination. It requires little effort to put the patient at ease. The following "Ten Commandments of Communication" for medical practices were published by Brown and Morley (1986):

I. Do not hurry; make the patient feel that he or she is the only one you have to think about at that moment.
II. Open each encounter with: "It's good to see you again," not, "Why are you here today?" Your contact with the patient should include a lot of eye contact and good, active listening.
III. Hold the opening encounter, no matter how brief, when the patient is dressed. That provides the opportunity to meet you initially on more comfortable terms. Walking in on a draped patient may make for quicker visits, but then people think of you as a doctor who is too busy to talk with them.
IV. Communicate with the patient on physically equal terms. Many physicians stand while talking with seated patients. This is seen as an authoritarian pose. This is how policemen interrogate suspects, towering over them, intimidating them physically and psychologically. An aware physician

does not do this. Instead, by placing two small chairs in each examining room, the examiner can sit close and be on the same level as the patient.

V.   Ask, "Is there anything else you are concerned about?" That gives the patient an opportunity to express any inner anxieties.

VI. Do not interrupt an encounter with a phone call unless absolutely necessary. "If he is that busy," thinks the patient, "maybe I should go elsewhere."

VII. End each meeting with, "It was good to see you. Thank you for coming." If the patient is sick, add, "I'm concerned about you, so call tomorrow and let me know how you are doing."

VIII. End each meeting by making sure that the patient understands what has been done, what has been found, and what the treatment will be. Many times, physicians assume that patients understand rather than making sure that they do.

IX. Provide oral and written instructions, and, when possible, back up those instructions with printed educational material, such as a brochure on high blood pressure.

X.   Listen to your patients. Pay particular attention to nonverbal cues, such as anger because of underlying fear.

PRESS RELEASES AND MEDIA OUTLETS

A clinic can use the media to get the practice name and or message to the public in a number of ways. The most effective advertising is that which cannot be paid for. A 30-second paid commercial slot on the evening news can cost from hundreds to thousands of dollars. A 2-minute story covering an aspect of the services offered by the clinic can be worth more than many paid commercial slots. A clinician may be fortunate enough to receive a call from a reporter who may be doing a story related to balance function, but through some simple planning the clinician can stimulate interest by means of a press release (Fig. 8–1). The press release must contain information regarding the 5 Ws—who, what, when, where, and why—and should be directed to a specific reporter (Solomon, 1991). To increase the odds that the press release will be used for a feature, the press release may be sent to more than one reporter as well as the assignment editor. The press release should make it clear that the information offered is timely and newsworthy. If a reporter calls to follow up, the clinician must be available for an interview at the convenience of the reporter. If the reporter is inconvenienced, he or she may decide to do a different story or, worse yet, call a competitor for an interview.

PAID ADVERTISEMENTS

Paid advertising is the most expensive method of getting a message to the public. Advertising can take many forms, and each form has its strengths and weakness. A simple method of establishing value of the various forms of paid advertising is to formulate an estimate of the "cost per potential patient." Simply dividing the

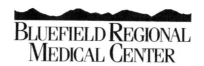

BLUEFIELD REGIONAL MEDICAL CENTER

September 23, 1998

Matt Hankins
Richlands News Press
Box 818
Richlands, VA 24641

Dear Matt:

Each year, millions of Americans visit their doctors for dizziness. In fact, dizziness is the third most frequent reason people seek medical attention, and the condition is especially prevalent in older adults. The condition challenges doctors and frustrates affected patients because it has many causes and, until now, few good treatments.

That's why we are proud to announce the establishment of the Bluefield Regional Centre for Dizziness and Balance Disorders. The center offers a unique team of specialists that works together to effectively diagnose and treat all types of dizziness and balance disorders.

I would personally like to invite you to an open house at the Bluefield Regional Center for Dizziness and Balance Disorders on Tuesday, September 29 at noon in Campus Building A, Suite 205. The Center's staff will be on hand to show you the new facilities and answer any questions you may have. We'll also provide media press packages, and lunch will be available.

I look forward to seeing you on Tuesday. In the meantime, please call me at 327-1150 if you have any questions.

Sincerely,

Tammy Halsey
Marketing and Public Relations Director

500 CHERRY STREET ● BLUEFIELD, WEST VIRGINIA, 24701 ● (304) 327-110

Figure 8–1. Sample press release.

cost of the advertisement by the number of potential patients reached will provide a "cost per" number that can be compared with other advertising media. Because vestibular disorders are much more common in older patients, placing advertisements in media that cater to this group will most likely provide a more cost-effective response. Print media such as newspapers and magazines tend to be more demographic specific, whereas television and the Yellow Pages are more generic.

The listings in the Yellow Pages provide an opportunity to gain new patients when a person is actively seeking out someone to provide the desired services. A caveat to a Yellow Page listing for patients with dizziness is the fact that potential patients may not know where to look in the phone book. In a rural area, simply placing an informative display ad under "Physicians" may be adequate. In a large urban area, a potential patient may not know what specialists handle dizziness.

Television advertising reaches the most people and probably has the greatest impact. On the negative side, television ads are quite costly both in terms of purchasing air time and in the production costs necessary for developing a professional-appearing, dignified spot. Additionally, production of these spots takes time; so they must be planned well in advance. Advertisements can be selectively placed on shows that are more geared toward an older population.

Radio advertising is less expensive than television and can also reach a targeted market (oldies or Big Band music stations will appeal to an older demographic). Radio provides for a short-message life and must be played repeatedly to get the message across. Because most patients do not sit by the radio with a pencil in hand, the listener must have additional access to information, such as address and phone number. If a Yellow Pages or newspaper advertisement is run concurrently, the listener can be referred to these for more information.

Newspaper advertising provides good exposure to the local market. Because most areas have small local as well as larger regional newspapers, the HCP can decide what format will provide the best type of exposure for the particular practice. Balance clinics are generally regional in nature, and so a larger regional newspaper may be more cost-effective. Weekly publications such as *The Senior Times* may have a much smaller distribution, but the lower cost to place the advertisement and the more specific readership make these publications attractive. Advertising agency specialists recommend using the following formula in designing a print ad for placement in a newspaper (Ogilvy, 1985; reprinted from Brown and Morley, 1986):

1. Place an illustration at the top of the page with a caption below it.
2. Print the copy in a serif typeface.
3. Set the copy in three columns 35 to 45 characters wide.
4. Start the copy with drop initials.
5. Print the copy in black ink on white paper.

See Appendix G for examples of newspaper ads promoting balance clinics.

Financial Aspects

As noted in Chapter 4, the cost of equipment needed for a comprehensive balance clinic can approach or exceed $200,000. The costs of some of the equipment have gradually decreased in the past few years, and it is debatable whether the more costly equipment (i.e., the rotational chair and Equitest) are necessary to perform reliable examinations. Nonetheless, the cost of equipment is an imposing and undeniable presence when considering expanding vestibular diagnostic facilities. These costs lead to the obvious questions: "How will I pay for the equipment?" and "Can I generate enough income to cover this expense with some profitability?"

Lease versus Purchase

Leasing high-technology medical equipment offers several advantages compared with direct purchase. Leasing can preserve working capital and minimize up-front expense, which can be important in the early stages of a practice. Most private practitioners find that there is an underutilization of their services in the first 1 to 3 years of practice. It takes time to build a reputation and a busy practice. Leasing allows one to spread the expense of equipment over a period of several years, thereby lowering the monthly payments.

Typically, some uncertainty exists as to whether the balance clinic will be successful. Leasing provides the option of using the equipment without owning it. If at the end of the lease term it is decided that the balance clinic is not a viable venture, the equipment can simply be returned to the leasing company. Depending on the level of confidence that the clinic will succeed, the leasing can be structured in a number of ways to best meet the needs of the clinic (leasing options to be discussed later).

Lease payments are usually considered a valid pretax expense and can be fully deducted. Purchase expense often must be depreciated over the useful life of the equipment; so, if the equipment is purchased by payment in full at the time of delivery, the practice may not be able to deduct all this expense from the annual financial statement. Finally, leasing guards against obsolescence. If at the end of the lease period the equipment is no longer adequate for the purposes of the clinic, it can be returned to the leasing company and a new lease for newer equipment can be obtained.

The obvious downside to leasing is the fact that the clinic does not own the equipment. A wise purchase can allow continued generation of income long after the equipment is paid for. One must also consider the additional expense of the fees imposed by the leasing company and compare those with current interest rates available by lending institutions. A financial adviser or accountant can help in comparing the relative costs of using working capital (which has the potential for earned interest) against the costs of leasing or borrowing money for equipment purchase.

Leasing Options

FAIR MARKET VALUE

At the end of the agreed lease period, the clinic has the option to purchase the equipment at its fair market value (defined as "what a willing buyer not under duress and a willing seller not under duress would agree to"). A method of determining fair market value should be agreed on before initiating the lease. This type of lease allows the lowest monthly payments.

TEN-PERCENT PURCHASE OPTION

At the end of the agreed lease period, the equipment can be purchased for 10% of its original cost, thereby allowing lower monthly payments than direct purchase, but it allows one to own the equipment at the end of the lease period if that is advantageous.

ONE-DOLLAR PURCHASE OPTION

At the end of the lease period, the equipment can be purchased for one dollar. Although the monthly payment would logically be no lower than direct purchase, there may be some tax advantages to leasing versus purchasing. Some taxing authorities view this type of lease as an intent to own; so tax treatment should be discussed with an accountant (www.keystoneleasing.com).

Reimbursement

The basic tenent of a successful business is that revenues must exceed expenses. As mentioned earlier in this chapter, income received from medical services is typically set by a third party and providers have little control over what they will be reimbursed for any particular service. Reimbursement rates can be researched before making a commitment to the purchase of equipment and other expenses associated with starting a balance clinic.

Diagnostic procedures used in the evaluation of vestibular patients are given code numbers so that they can be easily identified by third-party payers. These CPT (current procedural terminology) codes are five-digit numbers and are designated by the CPT Advisory Committee of the American Medical Association when there is agreement among the committee members that a new procedure has reached the status of widespread and justified use. Specific CPT codes for vestibular diagnostic procedures and descriptions are listed in Table 8–2.

All codes listed for vestibular diagnostic studies can be divided into the *professional component* and the *technical component*. The professional component is considered the value of the physician's input in interpreting the results of the procedure and providing a diagnosis as well as assuming the liability and associated malpractice expense. To indicate that the code is for the professional component only, a modifier (26) is placed after the five-digit code (e.g., 92541-26). The technical component reflects the value of the actual performance of the procedure and is indicated by the modifier TC (e.g, 92541-TC). When the same person is both performing and interpreting the procedure, no modifier is necessary (e.g., 92541). This is considered a *global component*.

Although each procedure and CPT code can be individually negotiated with managed care companies, many third-party payers are using the relative value unit (RVU) to determine the reimbursement for each particular procedure. The RVU scale is used to compare the relative value of one procedure compared with other medical procedures. The relative value of each procedure is dictated by the associated costs to the practitioner, which are intended to reflect "physician work" (knowledge and expertise required to perform the procedure), overhead

Table 8–2. CPT Codes for Vestibular Diagnostic Procedures

Code 92541 Nystagmus
Description: Spontaneous nystagmus test, including gaze and fixation nystagmus, with recording.
Spontaneous nystagmus tests document and measure the inability of the eyes to maintain a static position as a result of peripheral, central nervous system (CNS), or congenital abnormality. The tests are conducted with the eyes open and closed and in "eyes forward" as well as "eyes right" and "eyes left" positions.

Code 92542 Positional Nystagmus
Description: Positional nystagmus test, minimum of four positions, with recording.
These spontaneous nystagmus tests document and measure the inability of the eyes to maintain a static position when the head is in different positions. These tests are valuable in documenting and quantifying patient complaints of dizziness in certain situations or positions. Moreover, they are sometimes helpful to localize the abnormality as CNS or peripheral.

Code 92543 Calorics
Caloric vestibular test, each irrigation (binaural bithermal stimulation constitutes four tests), with recording. The caloric tests evaluate the viability of the peripheral end organs by stimulating them with warm and cool water while the patient's eyes are closed. The resulting dizziness and nystagmus are taken as an index of the viability of the organ. The eyes are then opened to evaluate the ability of the CNS to suppress visually inappropriate dizziness and nystagmus.

Code 92544 OKN or OPK
Optokinetic nystagmus test, bidirectional, foveal, or peripheral stimulation, with recording.
The optokinetic test documents and measures eye movements as the patients watches a series or targets moving simultaneously to the right and then to the left. The optokinetic mechanism is at work when the visual movement in one direction encompasses more than a single point.

Code 92545 Tracking or Smooth Pursuit
Oscillating tracking test, with recording.
This test evaluates the ability of the patient to keep a moving visual target registered on the fovea. The patient watches a light as it moves back and forth in a smooth pendular fashion. The computer computes the gain (target velocity divided by eye velocity) and compares the gain to age-matched norms.

Code 92546 VORTEQ: Active Head Rotation
Sinusoidal vertical axis rotational testing
This is a computerized test of the vestibular ocular reflex (VOR), the neural mechanism that keeps a visual image registered on the fovea during head movement. It evaluates the three functional components of the VOR system: the peripheral end organ, the vestibular nuclei of the brainstem, and the higher central vestibular connections. The test is accomplished by having the patient shake his or her head "no" and "yes" while wearing electro-oculography (EOG) electrodes that monitor eye position and a small angular velocity sensor that measures head velocity. From these data, the computer computes three characteristics of the VOR: gain (ratio of eye velocity to had velocity), phase (the number of

degrees by which the eye "misses" the target), and asymmetry (a comparison of gain moving right with gain moving left). This information in useful for evaluation patients with balance disorders.

Code 92546 Rotational Chair Test (Sinusoidal Harmonic Acceleration (SHA): Low Frequency)
Sinusoidal vertical axis rotational testing. This is a computerized slow harmonic acceleration rotation test to evaluate the integrity of the VOS. The test lasts 30 to 40 minutes and is run completely under computer control. This is an essential part in the evaluation of the dizzy patient because it reflects the relationship between natural head and eye movements involved in the balance mechanism.

Code 92547 Vertical Leads
Uses of vertical electrodes in any of all the above tests count as one additional test.

Code 92548 Computerized Dynamic Posturography
This is a computerized test that allows various systems that contribute to equilibrium to be assessed.

Reprinted with permission from Micromedical Technologies (www.micromedical.com).

(cost of supplies, equipment, and so forth), and professional liability (the difficulty factor and the cost of malpractice insurance). Medicare has adopted a system of "resource based" RVUs, not surprisingly referred to as RBRVS (resource-based relative value system). The RBRVS value is reduced if the procedure is performed in the hospital rather than the physician's office, presumably because the hospital provides the facility, staff, and equipment.

To arrive at a cash value for each of the RBRVS values, a conversion factor can be applied. As a baseline, Medicare's conversion factor falls between $31 and $38, depending on the geographic locality, with the national core conversion rate being $36.20 in 2002. For example, the code for "spontaneous nystagmus test" (92541) has an RVU for the professional component (92541-26) of 0.62. Multiply this value by the conversion factor ($36.20), and the professional component value for 92541 equals $22.44. The technical component (92541-TC) has an RVU of 1.27. Apply this to the conversion factor (again $36.20), and the technical component has a cash value of $45.97. The global component is the sum of the professional and technical components (RVU equals 0.62 plus 1.47 for a global RVU of 1.89). Applied to the conversion factor, the cash value of the total procedure is $68.41 (American Medical Association 2002). Medicare would then pay the provider $54.73 (80%), and the patient or supplemental insurance would be responsible for the remaining $13.68 (20%).

The CPT codes for vestibular rehabilitation (VR) would generally fall under the heading of "physical medicine." Physical medicine codes most applicable to VR are the following:

> 97530: "Therapeutic activities ... directed at loss or restriction of mobility, strength, balance and coordination"

97112: "Therapeutic procedure . . . to improve balance coordination, kinesthetic sense, posture and proprioception"

Diagnosis codes (ICD-9) for specific vestibular complaints such as vertigo and dysequilibrium, as well as for specific vestibular pathologies such as labyrinthitis and benign paroxysmal positional vertigo (BPPV), will not be accepted as appropriate diagnosis codes for billing the aforementioned codes applicable to VR. Covered diagnosis codes that are applicable to balance disorders and may benefit from VR include: 719.77 (difficulty walking), 781.2 (gait abnormality), and 781.9 (abnormal posture) (Medicare Newsletter, April 1997).

Medicare's reimbursement rates and conversion factors are considered on the lower end of the reimbursement spectrum and do not necessarily reflect the actual value or cost of these procedures. It is worthwhile to note these rates because most patients seeking services for vestibular disorders are older and Medicare is typically their primary provider. Because reimbursement and coding guidelines may change depending on the specific insurance carrier, the reader is advised to investigate local and current guidelines individually.

Once the reimbursement rate is established, the HCP can begin to estimate the volume of patients needed to generate enough revenue to cover the expenses of equipment, staff, and facility. It is hoped that a well-thought-out marketing strategy will result in a thriving balance clinic.

References

American Medical Association. (2002). *Medicare RBRVS: The physician's guide*.

Antman, E. M., Lau, J., Kupelnick, B., Mosteller, F., & Chalmers, T. C. (1992). A comparison of results of meta-analyses of randomized control trials and recommendations of clinical experts. Treatments for myocardial infarction. *JAMA*, *268*(2), 240–248.

Boyet, J. H., & Conn, H. P. (1991). *Workplace 2000*. New York: Plume.

Brown, S. W., & Morley, A. P. (1986). *Marketing strategies for physicians: A guide to practice growth*. Oradell, NJ: Medical Economics.

Health Care Consultants of America. (2000). *2000 Physician's fee & coding guide: A comprehensive coding & fee reference*. Augusta, GA: author.

Honrubia, V., Bell, T. S., Harris, M. R., Baloh, R. W., & Fisher, L. M. (1996). Quantitative evaluation of dizziness characteristics and impact on quality of life. *Am J Otol*, *17*(4), 595–602.

Hosford-Dunn, H., Dunn, D., & Harford, E. (1995). *Audiology business and practice management*. San Diego: Singular Publishing Group.

Keystone Leasing. Retrieved November 11, 20003, from www.keystoneleasing.com.

Medicare Newsletter. (April 1997). *Physical medicine and rehabilitation* (pp. 13–22). Columbus: Ohio, Nationwide Insurance.

Micromedical Technologies. Retrieved November 11, 2003, from www.micromedical.com.

Ogilvy, D. (1985). *Ogilvy on advertising*. New York: Vintage.

Solomon, R. J. (1991). *Clinical practice management*. Gaithersburg, MD: Aspen Publishers.

Staab, W. (2000). Marketing principals. In: H. Hosford-Dunn, R. J. Roeser, & M. Valente (Eds.), *Audiology practice management* (pp. 137–188). New York: Thieme Medical Publishers.

Appendixes

Appendix A Dizziness Handicap Inventory

P1. Does looking up increase your problem?

E2. Because of your problem do you feel frustrated?

F3. Because of your problem do you restrict your travel for business or recreation?

P4. Does walking down the aisle of a supermarket increase your problem?

F5. Because of your problems do you have difficulty getting into or out of bed?

F6. Does your problem significantly restrict your participation in social activities such as going out to dinner, movies, dancing, or parties?

F7. Because of your problem do you have difficulty reading?

P8. Does performing more ambitious activities like sports, dancing, and household chores such as sweeping or putting dishes away increase your problem?

E9. Because of your problems are you afraid to leave your home without having someone accompany you?

E10. Because of your problem have you been embarrassed in front of others?

P11. Do quick movements of your head increase your problem?

F12. Because of your problem do you avoid heights?

P13. Does turning over in bed increase your problem?

F14. Because of your problem is it difficult for you to do strenuous housework or yardwork?

E15. Because of your problem are you afraid people may think you are intoxicated?

F16. Because of your problem is it difficult for you to go for a walk by yourself?

P17. Does walking down a sidewalk increase your problem?

E18. Because of your problem is it difficult for you to concentrate?

F19. Because of your problem is it difficult for you to walk around your house in the dark?

E20. Because of your problem are you afraid to stay home alone?

E21. Because of your problem do you feel handicapped?

E22. Has your problem placed stress on your relationships with members of your family or friends?

E23. Because of your problem are you depressed?

F24. Does you problem interfere with your job or household responsibilities?

P25. Does bending over increase your problem?

"P" denotes physical subscale items, "E" denotes emotional subscale items, and "F" denotes functional subscale items. **Scoring: Yes, 4 points; Sometimes, 2 points; No, 0 points.**

Adapted from Jacobson GP, Newman CW, Hunter L, et al. (1991) *J Am Acad Audiol* 2, 253–260.

Appendix B   Motion Sensitivity Quotient

UNIVERSITY OF MICHIGAN VESTIBULAR TESTING CENTER HABITUATION TRAINING

NAME: _____   MRN: _____   AGE: _____   SEX: _____

DATE: _____

	INTENSITY	DURATION	SCORE
BASELINE SYMPTOMS			
1. SITTING → SUPINE			
2. SUPINE → LEFT SIDE			
3. →→ RIGHT SIDE			
4. SUPINE → SITTING			
5. LEFT HALLPIKE			
6. →→ SITTING			
7. RIGHT HALLPIKE			
8. →→ SITTING			
9. SITTING → NOSE TO LEFT KNEE			
10. SITTING → ERECT LEFT			
11. SITTING → NOSE TO RIGHT KNEE			
12. SITTING → ERECT RIGHT			
13. SITTING → HEAD ROTATION			
14. SITTING → HEAD FLEX. AND EXT.			
15. STANDING → TURN TO RIGHT			
16. STANDING → TURN TO LEFT			

INTENSITY: SCALE FROM 0 TO 5 (0=NO SX, 5=SEVERE SX)
DURATION: SCALE FROM 0 TO 3 (5-10 SEC=1 POINT, 11-30 SEC=2 POINTS, ≥30 SEC=3 POINTS)

TOTAL ____

MOTION SENSITIVITY QUOTIENT: $\dfrac{\text{\# POSITIONS} \times \text{SCORE}}{2048} \times 100 = $ _____

Reprinted with permission from Herdman, S. J. (2000). *Vestibular Rehabilitation*. Philadelphia: F.A. Davis Co.

Appendix C   Rehabilitation Exercises

Ankle sways

1. Have the patient stand on a firm surface with his or her feet shoulder distance apart, equal weight on both feet, and arms relaxed at the sides. Look straight ahead. This exercise may be performed with a target or in front of a mirror for extra visual reinforcement.
2. While he or she looks straight ahead, have the patient slowly shift his or her weight forward (toes) and backward (heels). Keep the amount of movement forward and back restricted to prevent bending at the hips. All movement should be at the ankles.
3. Next have the patient shift his or her weight from side to side, placing more weight first to the right side, then to the left. Again, prevent bending at the hips.
4. This exercise can be done with the eyes open, then closed. This exercise can also be done with the patient standing on a compliant surface such as a foam pad or cushion. Manipulation of these variables allows for sensory organization training.

Balance ball-bounce eyes fixed on target

1. Assist the patient to a sitting position on large physio ball. The patient's feet should be touching the floor with hands placed on the side of the ball.
2. Once the patient feels comfortable sitting on the ball, have the person slowly bounce on the ball while continuing to focus on the target.
3. After the patient is comfortable with this activity, hold a small object approximately 18 inches in front of the patient's eyes and tell him or her to focus on this object while resuming the bouncing action.

Balance beam

1. Patient is to place the right foot on the beam while the instructor provides assistance.
2. Assist the patient onto the beam and have him or her place the left foot in front of the right in a heel-to-toe pattern. The patient's eyes should be directed forward at all times.
3. Have the patient follow the path of the beam, keeping one foot in front of the other.
4. If needed, allow the patient to extend arms out to the side for balance.
5. This exercise can begin with the patient walking a tape line on the floor.

Balance-board exercise

1. Making sure that the feet are placed in the center of the board, assist the patient to a standing position on the balance board.
2. While keeping his or her body erect and preventing bending at the hips, have the patient gradually lean forward. (The board will move forward with the patient.)

3. Have the patient gradually lean back on the heels and come back to the center position. Have the patient continue leaning back further on his or her heels while the front of the board comes up. Have the patient lean forward without bending at the hips and come back to the center position.
4. Perform the exercise with movement from side to side.
5. Repeat the exercise but allow bending at the hips.

Ball circles

1. Have the patient stand with feet shoulder width apart, weight equal on both feet. Instruct the patient to hold a ball (or other soft object) with both hands, arms straight out from the body, and to keep his or her eyes on the ball at all times.
2. While keeping arms straight, the patient is to move the ball in a complete, smooth, and continuous circle. The patient is instructed to move the head as well as the eyes in this activity but is at all times to keep his or her eyes on the ball. Continue circling for a minimum of one minute in each direction.
3. The patient can also move the ball from side to side and up and down while keeping the eyes focused at all times. **If dizziness increases with this activity, the patient should stop movement until the feeling subsides, and then begin again.**
4. If the patient becomes very dizzy during this activity or is unsafe standing, this exercise can be done sitting in a chair, preferably one without arms.

Ball kicking

1. Instruct the patient that a ball will be slowly rolled toward him or her and that, on approach of the ball, the patient is to kick it back to the therapist with the side or top of their foot, whichever is most comfortable. Advise the patient that it is important to keep a wide stance and find their center of gravity before attempting to kick the ball.
2. Once the patient is standing comfortably and well balanced, gently roll the ball toward him or her. Alternate the foot used for kicking.
3. On having successfully completed this action and once the patient feels comfortable, instruct the patient to try taking two steps to the side before kicking the ball back.

Ball sitting

1. Carefully assist the patient into a sitting position on a physio ball. The feet should reach the floor comfortably.
2. Allow the patient to get his or her balance and to become as comfortable as possible.
3. The patient is to perform a rolling motion, first to the front and back and then side to side.
4. After the patient is comfortable with the ball, have the patient lift the legs off the ground while maintaining balance.

Ball toss

1. Instruct the patient that he or she is to attempt to catch the ball as it passes before him or her.
2. Stand to the side, a moderate distance from the patient, and gently toss a ball across the patient's front.
3. As the patient gains success in catching, toss the ball to different positions so that the patient must take additional action before catching the ball, such as taking a step, bending, stepping side to side, etc.

Bend and reach

1. Have the patient begin by standing in a wide, balanced position. Using proper lifting technique, the patient should pick up a ball from the floor and stand up. Then the patient should reach overhead to put the ball in the hands of the assistant.
2. This same procedure should be repeated for one minute, increasing in speed when possible.
3. The exercise should be repeated for one minute in the reverse order. Patient reaches up to take ball from assistant's hands and bends down to place the ball on the floor.
4. The patient should breathe appropriately and not hold his or her breath at any time.

Circle sways

1. Have the patient stand with the feet shoulder distance apart, arms resting at his or her sides.
2. The patient should breathe deeply and be encouraged to relax. The patient is to focus his or her thoughts on the feeling of the feet in contact with the floor.
3. Without bending at the hips, the patient is to practice swaying his or her body in a small circle. The patient is to sway forward repeatedly, to the right side, to the rear, to the left side, and forward again. A mirror may be used for extra visual reinforcement.
4. Have the patient gradually increase the size of the circle by moving his or her body farther each way, but without bending his or her hips or taking a step.
5. This exercise can be done with the eyes open and closed.

Crossover step

1. Have the patient stand near a wall with the feet slightly apart.
2. Instruct the patient to cross his or her right foot in front of the left, hold it there for 5 seconds, and then return the foot to its starting position.
3. Repeat this action with the left foot.
4. Have the patient repeat steps two and three repetitively for a specified number of times.

5. This exercise can be done with the eyes open and closed or in front of a mirror.

Face to knee

1. Have the patient start by sitting in an upright, comfortable position. Place each hand in a fist on each knee.
2. Slowly at first, have the patient bend over until the patient's face touches his or her fist. Bend down to the right, sweep over to the left, then sit up. Repeat bending down to the left, moving right, then sitting up.
3. Repeat, alternating, for a minimum of 1 minute making movements progressively faster if possible.

Foam sideways

1. Position the patient so that he or she is standing on one end of a foam floor mat and facing a wall, which will be used as a guide.
2. Making sure that the feet are pointing straight ahead (toward the wall), have the patient begin stepping sideways to the end of the mat and then return to the starting position.
3. Once the patient feels comfortable with this procedure have him or her perform the same action with eyes closed, first touching the wall, then without (increase use of proprioceptive input).

Foam walk

1. Position the patient so that he or she is standing at one end of a foam floor mat and facing the other end.
2. Have the patient walk at a comfortable pace using the stepping patterns and paths: forward, toe-toe, heel-heel, heel-heel to toe-toe, diagonal, and backward.
3. Instruct the patient to repeat each pattern a specified number of times.
4. This exercise can be done with the eyes open and closed, one hand on the wall.

Focus while turning head

1. Have the patient bring his or her index finger or a target to approximately 18 inches from the front of his or her nose (this can be done by taping a target to the wall).
2. While focusing on their target, have the patient turn his or her head from side to side for a minimum of one minute. Repeat the exercise moving the head up and down.
3. Gradually have the patient increase the speed of the head turns.

Note: This exercise can be done sitting if needed. When performed standing, the patient can initially assume a wide base of support. With improvements in standing balance, the base of support is gradually decreased.

Focus while turning head X 2

1. Have the patient hold a business card in front of himself or herself so that he or she can read it. The patient should move his or her head and the card side to side *in opposite directions* while keeping eyes on the card.
2. The head should be moved as quickly as possible, keeping the words or letter in focus. Continue this for 1-2 minutes without stopping.
3. Repeat this exercise moving the head up and down.

Note: This exercise can be done while sitting if needed. When performed standing, the patient can initially assume a wide base of support. With improvements in standing balance, the base of support is gradually decreased.

Foot work

1. This exercise can be performed sitting or standing, whichever is more comfortable and safe for the patient. A collection of objects of different size and texture should be presented to the patient.
2. The patient is instructed to feel the object with his or her foot and describe the texture and size. If the object can be picked up, the patient should attempt to do so with his or her foot.
3. It is important that the patient concentrate on the sensation and location of the object on the foot. Each foot should be presented several objects.

Hand-to-hand ball toss

1. Have patient sit in a chair preferably without arms.
2. Using a tennis or other small rubber ball, have the patient toss the ball from hand to hand above his or her eye level.
3. As the patient feels comfortable with this activity while sitting, have him or her do the same ball tossing while standing in a stable, centered stance.

Head circles

1. Have the patient begin moving the head in a circular motion with the eyes open.
2. Specifically, the patient is to first place his or her chin on their chest, then left ear on his or her left shoulder, move his or her head directly across to, right ear on right shoulder, and finally return the chin to his or her chest. Do not have the patient bend the head backward.
3. Assist the patient in making this motion as fluid as possible for a minimum of 1 minute.
4. After the patient becomes comfortable with this activity, have him or her reverse the direction of rotation.
5. Repeat the exercise in both directions with eyes closed.

Note: This exercise can be done sitting if needed. When performed standing, the patient can initially assume a wide base of support. With improvements in standing balance, the base of support is gradually decreased.

Head movements

1. While keeping the trunk still, have the patient quickly turn his or her head and look to the right, then turn and look to the left, and then return to center returning to the forward looking position. Have the patient maintain this forward looking position for 5 seconds. Repeat for 1 minute.
2. Have the patient perform the exercise, moving his or her head up and down.
3. This exercise can also be done with the eyes closed.

Note: This exercise can be done sitting if needed. When performed standing, the patient can initially assume a wide based stance. With improvements in standing balance, the base of support is gradually decreased.

Imaginary target

1. Have the patient fixate on a visual target directly in front of him or her, close the eyes, and rotate the head in one direction, imagining that he or she is still looking directly at the target. After the head rotation has stopped, the eyes are opened. The eyes should still be held on the target.
2. Repeat in the opposite direction. The patient should be as accurate as possible. Vary the speed and the amount (stopping point) of head rotation.
3. Repeat the exercise, but move the head up and down.
4. Practice for 5 minutes, stopping if necessary.

Moving saccades

1. The patient can start this exercise sitting if necessary but should advance to a standing progression as soon as possible. Place two targets at eye level, arm's length away, and slightly greater than shoulder width apart.
2. The patient starts with the head rotated approximately 40 degrees to the right with gaze directed at the right visual target. With the head stationary, gaze is shifted with a saccade to fixate on the visual target on the left, followed by the patient rotating the head to face the left target.
3. The movements are then repeated in the opposite direction. Patients are instructed to perform these movements as quickly as possible, while keeping the visual target in focus. The exercise should be performed for a minimum of 1 minute.

Obstacle course

1. Set up an obstacle course using chairs, pillows, trash can, and whatever else might be readily available. Some of the objects should be small enough that the patient can step over them and still see them so that they can be walked around.
2. The patient is then instructed to walk the obstacle course in a specified route or pattern.
3. As the patient progresses, have him or her pick up and carry the smaller objects.

4.   In time, change the course so that it does not become routine. To add difficulty, the clinician may toss a ball to the patient to catch as he or she walks.

One-leg stand

1.   Have the patient stand on one leg, with his or her back to a padded corner for safety, for 30 seconds.
2.   This activity should be done 10 times on each leg.
3.   This exercise can be done with the eyes open and closed.

Roll body against wall

1.   Have the patient stand with his or her back against a wall. Instruct him or her to take the right shoulder off the wall and turn to the left until the front of his or her body is against the wall.
2.   In a similar manner have the patient take his or her left shoulder off the wall and turn to the left until his or her back is again against the wall.
3.   Have the patient continue steps one and two until he or she has moved down the wall to its end. At this point instruct the patient to stop and regain balance.
4.   Have the patient return to the starting position and repeat this activity for a specified number of times.
5.   This exercise can be done with the eyes open and closed.

Saccades

1.   Have the patient hold a small index card in each hand, level with the eyes, at arms length, and about 18 inches apart.
2.   Keeping his or her head still and without stopping between cards, have the patient look quickly from one card to the other. Have the patient perform this action for 1 to 2 minutes.
3.   Repeat the exercise having the patient perform the same action but in a vertical direction.

Note: This exercise can be done sitting if needed. When performed in standing, the patient can initially assume a wide base of support. With improvements in standing balance, the base of support is gradually decreased.

Sit to stand

1.   Have the patient begin by sitting in an unarmed chair (arms can be used if needed).
2.   The patient should rise quickly, using only his or her legs, looking straight ahead. He or she should remain standing for 5 seconds or until any dizziness is gone.
3.   Next the patient should sit back down into the chair in a controlled but rapid manner. Do not let him or her just drop into the chair. The patient

should use his or her legs to control the descent. He or she should remain sitting for 5 seconds or until any dizziness is gone.

4. This exercise can be done with two chairs facing each other. The patient should stand, turn around, and sit in the opposite chair.
5. This exercise can be repeated with the eyes closed.
6. This exercise should not be performed on patients with postural or orthostatic hypotension.

Sit to supine

1. Have the patient sit on foam or a padded platform that he or she can fully recline on and place a pillow under the patient's knees.
2. Instruct the patient to turn his or her head to the desired side.
3. Have the patient lie down as rapidly as possible so that he or she is flat and keeping the head turned.
4. Have the patient stay in this position for as long as the symptoms last (or for 15 seconds if no symptoms).
5. Have the patient sit up as rapidly as possible.
6. Once sitting, wait until symptoms again subside (or 30 seconds if no symptoms).
7. Repeat the exercises with the patient for the desired number of times.

Sitting on a chair/stool

1. Have the patient sit quietly and without moving on a firm surface such as a chair or stool, breathe deeply a few times, and relax.
2. Instruct the patient to concentrate on the sensation of sitting in the chair or stool. A mirror may be used for extra visual reinforcement.
3. Next have the patient close his or her eyes for 10 seconds and again to concentrate on the sensation of his or her body sitting.

Standing

1. Have the patient stand in front of a long mirror hands, at his or her sides, feet shoulder-width apart, head up, shoulders back, and looking straight ahead. Have the patient notice his or her posture and instruct him or her to maintain this posture throughout the exercise. Ask the patient to concentrate on not swaying and to stand still for 1 minute.
2. Have the patient maintain this same stance but look straight ahead at a target on the wall. Maintain this position for 1 minute.
3. Progressively narrow the base of support (move feet closer 1 inch at a time) from feet apart, to feet together, to a semiheel-to-toe position, to heel to toe (one foot in front of the other). Do the exercises first with the arms outstretched, then with arms close to the body, and then with arms folded across the chest. Hold each position for 30 seconds, and then move to the next most difficult position. Alternate between mirror and target.
4. Repeat above with head bent forward 30 degrees and then back 30 degrees.

5. Repeat the basic standing exercise with eyes closed, at first intermittently and then continuously, instructing the patient to make an effort to visualize mentally his or her surroundings.

6. All these exercises can also be performed while standing on a foam mat or other uneven surface.

7. Be sure to maintain a position near the patient to assist him or her if needed, especially during the time when he or she has eyes closed. Some patients may need these instructions given in sections because they will try to do too much too soon if not directed. The patient should only move on when he or she can successfully complete the previous section.

Stepping patterns

1. This exercise uses numbered squares arranged in a pattern on the floor.

2. Instruct the patient to stand behind a base line, to tap the designated foot on the specified card as its number is called forth, and then return the foot to the starting position.

3. Tell the patient which foot to use and call out the 2, 3, or 4 numbers in a row.

Targets

1. Choose three targets that are at eye level, one directly in front of the patient, one to the extreme right, and the other to the extreme left.

2. Have the patient, turning only the head, look at the target to the left, then the one at center, and then to the target located to the right. Focus on each target.

3. Have the patient repeat this activity for 1 minute without stopping.

4. When the patient is ready, have the same exercise repeated except he or she is to stop at each target to focus.

5. This exercise can also be done horizontally or vertically.

Note: This exercise can be done sitting if needed. When performed standing, the patient can initially assume a wide base of support. With improvements in standing balance, the base of support is gradually decreased.

Trace the alphabet

1. Position the patient near a wall or counter so that he or she has something to hold on to if it becomes necessary.

2. Have the patient trace the first 10 letters of the alphabet on the floor with his or her foot. Once completed have the patient repeat the tracing procedure with the other foot.

3. As the patient's proficiency improves with step 2, have him or her trace all the letters of the alphabet.

Tracking exercise

1. Give the patient a small index card with several words written on it. Instruct the patient to hold the card about 18 inches in front of his or her eyes.
2. While keeping their head still and following the card only with his or her eyes, have the patient slowly move the card horizontally to the right, to the left, and back to center. Have the patient perform this action for a minimum of 1 minute.
3. As the patient progresses in ability, have him or her move the arm at faster and faster speeds until no longer able to read the words. Remember, the patient is to keep the head still during this exercise and follow the card only with the eyes.
4. This exercise should also be done with vertical and diagonal movement.

Note: This exercise can be done sitting if needed. When performed standing, the patient can initially assume a wide base of support. With improvements in standing balance, the base of support is gradually decreased.

Tracking/VOR interaction

1. While the patient is standing on an uneven or movable surface, (e.g., trampoline, vestibular board, foam mat) have him or her focus on an object that you move in front of the field of vision. Instruct the patient to maintain his or her balance while focusing on the object.
2. As the patient becomes proficient in this activity, vary the exercise by moving the object in a vertical or diagonal motion.

Trampoline ankle sway

1. Position the patient on the trampoline so that his or her feet are shoulder width apart, with equal weight on both feet, arms relaxed at their side, and looking straight forward at a target.
2. Have the patient slowly and carefully shift his or her weight forward and then backward. All movement should be at the ankles, and the patient should not be allowed to bend at the hips.
3. Next have the patient shift his or her weight from side to side, placing more weight first on the right side and then on the left. Again, do not permit the patient to bend at the hips.
4. This exercise can be repeated with the eyes closed.

Trampoline circle sway

1. Assist the patient to the center of the trampoline with his or her feet shoulder distance apart.
2. Relax the patient by having him or her breathe deeply and slowly expel the air.
3. Have the patient slowly sway his or her body in small circles. Instruct and help him or her sway forward, to the right side, to the rear, to the left side

and forward again. This should be performed without the patient bending at the hips.

4. As the patient progresses in his or her ability have him or her gradually increase the size of the circle while making sure not to bend at the hips or take a step.
5. This exercise can be performed with the eyes closed.

Trampoline walk

1. Instruct the patient to step slowly up onto the trampoline, and provide assistance when necessary. The patient is to keep his or her head up and eyes focused on a specified, fixed object located at eye ievel.
2. Beginning with small steps at first, the patient is to increase gradually the stepping height and speed until he or she is almost marching.
3. Once the patient feels comfortable with the stepping motion, have him or her continue to step and then march with eyes closed.

Walk stop

1. Have the patient begin walking approximately 10 steps at a good pace and then have him or her stop abruptly at your command. Allow the patient sufficient time to regain balance.
2. Have the patient repeat this activity a specified number of times.

Walking with eyes closed

1. Before having the patient perform this exercise, have him or her walk the length of the room next to a wall with their eyes open. Ask him or her to pay attention and get used to the surface.
2. Standing a little away from the wall, have the patient extend his or her arms out so that the fingertips are lightly touching the wall.
3. Using the wall as a guide, have the patient begin walking along the wall with his or her eyes closed and head up. The patient should attempt to imagine a straight line as he or she walks.
4. If the patient at anytime feels off balance or likely to fall, he or she is to open his or her eyes. Only after the patient feels that he or she has regained balance is he or she to begin again.

Walking with head turns

1. Instruct the patient to begin walking at normal speed (Walk next to him or her to assure safety).
2. Have the patient turn his or her head to the right and left as they walk (about every three steps).
3. Instruct him or her to try to focus on different objects while walking.
4. Gradually he or she should move the head faster and more often.
5. Have the patient repeat this activity for a minimum of 2 minutes.

This exercise should also be performed with head movements up and down and diagonal.

Walking with turns

1. Have the patient walk in a large circle but gradually make smaller and smaller turns. Be sure to have the patient make circles in each direction.
2. When circles are relatively small, have the patient take five steps and turn around to the right (180 degrees) and keep walking. Take five more steps, turn to the left (180 degrees) and keep walking. Repeat 5 times, rest, and repeat the entire sequence.

Appendix D   Example of a Patient Flowchart for a Multispecialty Balance Disorders Clinic

Prior to day one: Information packet and questionnaire sent to patient with instructions to fill out questionnaire **prior to** arriving for appointment.

Day 1

1. History
2. Screening exams: nystagmus, head thrust, positional tests, hyperventilation
3. Audiometric evaluation
4. Summary report of history and screening test results

Medical Examination

1. Routine ENT exam
2. Cranial nerve exam
3. Review medications and instruct the patient about which medications to cease for evaluation
4. Order appropriate lab studies
5. Listen for bruits
6. Check for postural hypotension
7. Audiology and otolaryngology consult, and make recommendations for additional studies.
8. If vestibular evaluation is not indicated, the patient may be referred to another specialist or back to the referring physician

Day 2

Vestibular Evaluation: Scheduled with vestibular technician and senior audiologist

1. Calibration
2. Spontaneous, gaze, and positional (Hallpike's and static) nystagmus test
3. Rotational tests (active head rotation or rotary chair)
4. Oculomotor tests
5. Calorics
6. Auditory evoked potentials: ABR or EcoG in suspected Hydrops patients.

Physical Therapy

1. Posturography: sensory organization test
2. Assessment of strength and sensation of the lower extremities
3. Assessment of gait, weight shifts, reach test (limits of stability)
4. Handwritten notes faxed back to otolaryngology asap

5. Schedule patients for follow up in 1 week
    Compilation of results; dictate report, including impressions and recommendations

Day 3

1. Patient returns for consultation and review of test results
2. Depending on findings:
    a. Canalith repositioning (CRM): may do on day one if obvious
    b. Schedule for initial therapy session
    c. Medical consult regarding medications and bloodwork if needed
    d. Discuss referral to another specialty if indicated

Physical therapy

1. Therapy schedule determined on an individual basis: consider severity of symptoms, critical period of compensation, motivation, distance, and family support.
2. Final session: Outcome measures and report to balance clinic and/or referring physician. Discuss referral to another specialty if indicated

Follow-up

CRM: one week follow-up
Hydrops (Meniere's) regimen: 6-week follow-up
All patients seen for screening are called at 4 weeks to check on symptoms and outcomes of recommendations.

Appendix E   Sample of Newsletter to Physicians

BLUE RIDGE
ENT & Facial Surgery Center, Inc.
Hearing & Balance Clinic
Since 1983

OTOLARYNGOLOGY	AUDIOLOGY
Dr. Lee Smith	Alan L. Desmond, MS, CCC-A
Dr. Robert Jones	Pamela Given, MA, CCC-A
Dr. Brian Collie	Shanna Lahr, M.eD, CCC-A

100 New Hope Road • Medical Arts Building Princeton, West Virginia 487-3407 • 487-2487 (Audiology)	BRMC Campus • 210 Cherry Street, #205 Bluefield, West Virginia 324-2954

BENIGN POSITIONAL VERTIGO

Benign Paroxysmal Positional Vertigo (BPPV) is by far the most common cause of episodic vertigo. Patients typically report brief episodes (less than one minute) of intense vertigo, usually brought on by lying down, rolling over in bed, or tilting their head back. BPPV is a mechanical dysfunction of the inner ear, and does not usually represent an ongoing disease process. It is relatively easily diagnosed and treated. BPPV does not respond to medication, but rather is most effectively treated by canalith repositioning procedures.

BPPV is believed to be a result of small calcium carbonate crystals, which have become dislodged from the otolith structure, settling in the posterior semi-circular canal. These crystals, known as otoconia, cause no problem until the patient moves in a manner stimulating the offending semi-circular canal. The otoconia then begin moving, causing abnormal stimulation of the motion sensor in the affected ear. While the otoconia is in motion (typically 15 to 45 seconds) the patient is experiencing conflicting signals from the two labyrinths.

BPPV can be diagnosed by performing the Hallpike (also known as the Nylen or Barany) maneuver. If this maneuver makes the patient vertiginous, the eyes should simultaneously be inspected for nystagmus. The direction of the nystagmus allows for identification of the specific offending canal. Once this has been accomplished, the patient can be treated. The Canalith Repositioning Maneuver (CRM) is a relatively new procedure, and is still available only in a minority of Otolaryngologists offices. The CRM is a simple, non-invasive procedure designed to move the otoconia out of the offending semi-circular canal. The success rate of this procedure is over 90% when performed by an experienced clinician.

A LOW COST OPTION FOR BETTER HEARING

It is well known that only about 20% of patients with significant hearing loss wear hearing aids. There are a number of reasons for this. Many hearing impaired patients are unaware of the severity of their hearing loss, as the problem is usually more obvious to friends and family members. Some don't believe hearing aids will help based on bad past expe-
(continued on page 2)

CLINICAL INDICATORS FOR TONSILLECTOMY AND ADENOIDECTOMY
Reprint from the American Academy of Otolaryngology – 1998 Clinical Indicators Compendium

Patient Information

Removal of tonsils and/or adenoids is one of the most frequently performed throat operations. It has proven to be a safe, effective surgical method to resolve breathing obstruction, throat infections, and manage recurrent childhood ear disease. Pain fol-
(continued on page 3)

Appendix F   Referral Slip That Can Be Sent to Potential Referring Physicians

Blue Ridge Hearing and Balance Clinic
"A Sensible Way to Better Hearing and Balance"

510 Cherry St. #205	100 New Hope Road #19
Bluefield, WV 24701	Princeton, WV 24740
Phone: (304) 324-2954	Phone: (304) 487-2487
Fax: (304) 324-2955	Fax: (304) 431-3367

Referring Physician _____ Date _____

This will introduce my patient

_____

For: ❏ Diagnosis Only   ❏ Diagnosis and Treatment

Regarding: ❏ Hearing Problem   ❏ Balance Problem   ❏ Tinnitus
              ❏ Speech Problem   ❏ Middle Ear Problem   ❏ Other _____

Appointment: ❏ Monday   ❏ Tuesday   ❏ Wednesday   ❏ Thursday   ❏ Friday

        Date _____ at _____ A.M.
                                                P.M.

Physician Signature _____ UPIN # _____

If referring for balance evaluation please complete remainder of form.

Please evaluate this patient for complaints of dizziness or balance difficulties. The following general medical information and history is intended to allow more thorough evaluation of this patient.

History:

_____ Stroke   _____ Diabetes

_____ Neurologic Disease   _____ Peripheral Neuropathies

_____ Visual Problems   _____ Circulatory Problems

Please have patient bring ALL current medications to their appointment.
*We will provide an analysis of possible side effects and interactions for this list.

We appreciate any medical records that may assist us in our evaluation.

Certain medications can influence the body's response to vestibular tests, thus giving false and misleading results. If possible, please instruct your patient to refrain from taking the following types of medication 24 hours prior to their appointment:

ALCOHOL, ANALGESICS/NARCOTICS, ANTIHISTAMINES, ANTI-EMETIC or ANTI-VERTIGO MEDS, SEDATIVES OR TRANQUILIZERS

Physical Therapy evaluation if indicated   _____ OKAY   _____ CALL FIRST
Neurologic evaluation if indicated?   _____ OKAY   _____ CALL FIRST

(map on back)

Appendix G   Samples of Newspaper Advertisements

Sample 1

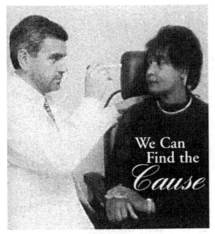

Each year millions of Americans visit their doctor for dizziness.

Unfortunately, half of all patients with this condition do not find the reason for their symptoms and only a third receive beneficial treatment. That's because dizziness can have many causes and pinpointing the exact reason for the condition and providing effective treatment can be difficult.

That's why we have established the Bluefield Regional Center for Dizziness and Balance Disorders. Our team of medical experts are trained and experienced in finding the specific causes of dizziness. Plus, our treatment strategies have proven highly effective for the majority of patients.

We Can Find the *Cause* of Your Dizziness.

If you or someone you love suffers from dizziness, call the Bluefield Regional Center for Dizziness and Balance Disorders.

We can help restore your health and your quality of life.

Bluefield Regional Center for Dizziness and Balance Disorders

BLUEFIELD REGIONAL
MEDICAL CENTER

Campus Building A, Suite 205
Bluefield, WV   (304) 324-2954

Sample 2

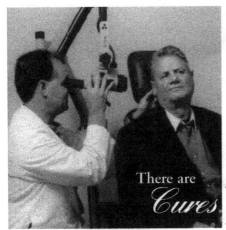

Dizziness is the third most frequent reason people seek medical attention.

Dizziness is the third most frequent reason people seek medical attention. Unfortunately, the condition challenges doctors and frustrates patients because it has many causes, and until now, few good treatments.

Helping doctors and their patients pinpoint the causes of dizziness and finding effective cures is the reason we have established the Bluefield Regional Center for Dizziness and Balance Disorders. All the members of our medical team are experts in the field of dizziness and balance disorders. They work together to find the cause, and the cure, for each patient who suffers from dizziness.

There are *Cures* for Your Dizziness.

If you or someone you love suffers from dizziness, call Bluefield Regional Center for Dizziness and Balance Disorders. We can help restore your health and your quality of life.

Bluefield Regional Center for Dizziness and Balance Disorders

BLUEFIELD REGIONAL
MEDICAL CENTER

Campus Building A, Suite 205
Bluefield, WV
(304) 324-2954

Sample 3

Falls are the leading cause of injury in older adults.

There are many factors that can contribute to falling. For example, as you age your balance system becomes less efficient. In fact, falls account for over 200,000 hip fractures each year in the United States.

The experts at Bluefield Regional Center for Dizziness and Balance Disorders are trained and experienced in pinpointing the factors that contribute to poor balance. Plus, we specialize in providing solutions that minimize your risk for falls.

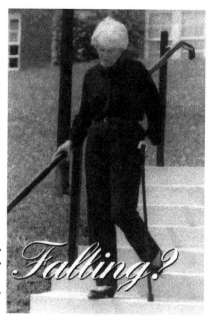

Afraid of

Don't become the victim of a fall. Call the Bluefield Regional Center for Dizziness and Balance Disorders. We can help you maintain your good health and your quality of life.

BLUEFIELD REGIONAL MEDICAL CENTER

Campus Building A, Suite 205
Bluefield, WV
(304) 324-2954

Bluefield Regional Center for Dizziness and Balance Disorders

Glossary

Acoustic reflex: Measures contraction of the stapedius and tensor tympani muscles in response to loud sounds.

Agoraphobia: An abnormal fear of being in open or public places (*Webster's*, 1976).

Ataxia: Defective muscular coordination.

Auditory brain stem response (ABR): The recording of electrical potentials generated by auditory stimulation of the cochlea. Frequently used as a screening method for auditory nerve function.

Barotrauma: Injury to the middle ear caused by a marked difference in middle ear pressure and the surrounding pressure, as in diving.

Benign paroxysmal positional vertigo (BPPV): A brief, violent vertiginous episode occurring within seconds after a change in head position. BPPV is the most common cause of episodic vertigo.

Caloric stimulation: The introduction of warm or cool air or water into the external ear canal to stimulate the vestibular system.

Dysequilibrium: A sense of unsteadiness or imbalance typically exacerbated by movement or environmental influences.

Effusion: The escape of fluid into a body cavity or tissue.

Electronystagmography (ENG): The recording of eye movements, especially nystagmus, by detecting changes in the electric potential between the cornea and the retina of the eyeball. It uses electrodes placed on the skin near the eyes, usually one pair of electrodes to monitor horizontal movement and another pair to monitor vertical movement.

Electro-oculography: The recording and study of eye movements.

Geotropic nystagmus: Refers to the direction of nystagmus beats relative to head position. Geotropic nystagmus beats toward the earth. Ageotropic nystagmus beats away from the earth.

Labyrinthectomy: Surgical removal or destruction of the labyrinth of the ear

Meniere's disease (endolymphatic hydrops): Recurrent vertigo, fluctuating sensory–neural hearing loss in one ear, and tinnitus in the same ear caused by increased pressure in the membranous labyrinth.

Nystagmus: Involuntary back-and-forth or rotary movements of the eyeball, named for the fast movement when fast and slow movements alternate.

Oscillopsia: Apparent movement of the visual scene resulting from involuntary retinal slip in acquired ocular oscillations or deficient vestibular ocular reflex.

Otalgia: Ear pain.

Otoconia: Calcium carbonate crystals normally found on the utricle and saccule; displacement of these crystals can result in benign paroxysmal positional vertigo.

Peripheral neuropathy: Impairment of sensation in the extremities frequently associated with diabetes and other circulatory diseases.

Proprioceptive: Pertaining to the awareness of touch and of body movement and position.

Pure-tone audiometry: The patient is placed in a sound-treated booth and asked to respond to tonal stimulus that varies in frequency (pitch) and intensity (loudness). These tones are presented through headphones (air conduction) and an oscillator (bone conduction). If there is a significant difference between air and bone conduction scores (air–bone gap), a conductive loss exists.

Rollover: Excessive (20% or more) decline in speech understanding as intensity is increased.

Sensitivity: The proportion of people who truly have a specific disease and are so identified by the test.

Somatosensory: See *proprioceptive.*

Specificity: The proportion of people who are truly free from a specific disease and are so identified by the test.

Speech recocognition tests: Scored as the percent repeated correctly of a list of monosyllabic words presented at varying intensities.

Speech recocognition threshold (SRT): The faintest sound level at which a patient can understand and repeat speech at a 50% accuracy level. This test is useful in verifying the accuracy of pure-tone results.

Tinnitus: Ringing or other sounds in the ear, usually heard only by the affected person.

Tympanometry: A measure of tympanic membrane (TM) integrity and mobility that provides information regarding middle ear effusion, TM perforation, and eustachian tube dysfunction.

Vertigo: A sensation of rotating, either of oneself (subjective vertigo) or of one's surroundings (objective vertigo).

Vestibular ocular reflex (VOR): Serves to maintain clear vision during head movement.

Although terms such as *vestibular rehabilitation, vestibular adaptation, vestibular compensation,* and *vestibular habituation* seem to be used interchangeably in the literature, important distinctions can be made. For the purposes of this book, we use the following definitions:

Vestibular rehabilitation refers to the process of training the patient in the techniques for recovery from vestibular weakness. *Rehabilitation* in general is defined as the process of "putting back in good condition, bringing or restoring to a normal or optimal state of health by medical treatment and … therapy" (*Webster's*, 1976).

Vestibular adaptation refers to the response of the central nervous system to asymmetrical peripheral vestibular afferent activity and resulting sensory conflicts. This implies a gradual decrease in neuronal response to constant abnormal stimuli (Curthoys & Halmagyi, 1996).

Vestibular compensation encompasses the entire repertoire of strategies used by the patient to reduce symptoms and improve overall balance function and stabilize gaze. This includes neuronal adaptation of the vestibular ocular reflex (VOR), sensory substitution, and alternative predictive and cognitive strategies used to overcome the symptoms of vestibular deficit (Zee, 1994).

Vestibular habituation is "the long term reduction in a neurologic response to a particular stimulus that is facilitated by repeated exposure to the stimulus. In the vestibular system, the unpleasant response is usually a vertiginous sensation, often associated with nausea, in response to certain head movements" (Shepard & Telian, 1996). In this context, vestibular rehabilitation involves maximizing vestibular compensation and promoting the learning and formation of habits (habituation) to promote reduction of symptoms and enhance postural and gaze stability.

References

Curthoys, I. S., & Halmagyi, G. M. (1996). How does the brain compensate for vestibular lesions? In Baloh, R.W., & Halmagyi, G. M. (Eds.), *Disorders of the vestibular system* (pp. 145–154). New York: Oxford University Press.

Guralnik, D. B. (Ed.). (1976). *Webster's new world dictionary.* Cleveland, OH: William Collins & World Publishing.

Shepard, N. T., & Telian, S. A. (1996). *Practical management of the balance disorder patient.* San Diego: Singular Publishing Group.

Thomas, C. L. (Ed.). (1997). *Taber's cyclopedic medical dictionary.* Philadelphia: F.A. Davis.

Zee, D. S. (1994). Vestibular adaptation. In Herdman, S. J. (Ed.). *Vestibular rehabilitation* (pp. 68–79). Philadelphia: F.A. Davis.

Index

Page numbers followed by f and t represent figures and tables, respectively. Page numbers in italics represent glossary entries.